D0904072

Determinants
of the
Nurse-Patient Relationship

Determinants *of the* Nurse-Patient Relationship

By

GERTRUD UJHELY

Associate Professor; Director, Graduate Program, Psychiatric Nursing; Adelphi University, School of Nursing

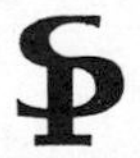

SPRINGER PUBLISHING COMPANY, INC.
NEW YORK

ALBRIGHT COLLEGE LIBRARY

By the same author:

The Nurse and Her Problem Patients

Copyright © 1968

200 Park Avenue South • New York, N.Y. 10003

SPRINGER PUBLISHING COMPANY, INC.

Library of Congress Catalog Card Number: 68-23551

Printed in U.S.A.

ALBRIGHT COLLEGE LIBRARY

610.696
U33d

139026

To the memory of

CLAUDIA AND VERA

Preface

I first thought of writing this book in the winter of 1962. Nursing students and practitioners had repeatedly asked me questions that related to problems they encountered in adapting the general principles of the nurse-patient relationship to specific situations. It seemed to me, therefore, that it was (and is) not enough to teach "interpersonal relations and sociopsychiatric concepts" as such, and not enough to remind the students of their existence in the various subdisciplines of nursing, but that nurses need additional guidelines for application of these concepts to the recurrent variables that they are likely to encounter in their practice. Some of these variables are inherent in the nurse and others in the patient as a person or in his condition; still others depend upon the situation within which the nurse-patient relationship takes place.

Discussion with other faculty members at the College of Nursing at Rutgers, the State University of New Jersey, where I was working at that time, and with teachers of psychiatric nursing and "integrators of sociopsychiatric concepts" from other schools corroborated my impressions. The literature of the past five years indicates that I have not been alone in attempting to place the nurse-patient relation in a framework that would permit an easy transition from concept to a specific case.

The book is directed primarily to two groups: 1) Students in preservice nursing programs who are encouraged to use principles as bases for their clinical practice; 2) graduate nurses who are looking for guidelines that might help them to meet the challenges of diverse clinical situations.

I hope, furthermore, that faculty groups in schools of nursing, particularly in basic collegiate programs, might consider the structure and content of the book as an example of how interpersonal aspects—and perhaps all aspects—of a nursing curriculum can be organized. Finally, there may be graduate students in nursing who may wish to consider some of the assertions made in the book as hypotheses that they will test through research.

Although I have made relatively little mention of the nurse's relationship to members of her own or other disciplines, I do not consider these topics unimportant. Rather I felt that a lengthy consideration of intra- and interdisciplinary relationships might cloud the purpose and content of this book. I also felt that clarity about her professional focus and its applications would, in itself, aid the nurse in her communication with peers.

The book deals with many variables that affect the nurse-patient relationship, but does not aim to be all-inclusive. The number of factors that may influence the way the nurse could and should relate to her clients is infinite. If too many of these factors were enumerated, their number alone would have obliterated my purpose of presenting general categories of factors and guidelines for dealing with them. It is hoped that each reader of this book will fit into the framework which I have presented examples drawn from her own experience.

The point of view underlying the book does not represent one particular school of thought but rather my own synthesis of various sources. The language has been kept simple so that the book may be read and understood by the beginning student in nursing, but many items among the suggested readings are by no means simple.

In order to avoid too frequent repetition of the terms "nurse" and "patient" I have, here, as in my other book, *The Nurse and Her Problem Patients*, designated the pronoun "she" for the nurse and the pronoun "he" for the patient.

The book should not be taken as a final and definitive statement but rather as one person's attempt to tie together important determinants of the nurse-patient relationship. It is not the first such attempt, nor will it be the last. If the book will become a guide for some of its readers and a take-off point for discussion and dissent for others, it will have amply served its purpose.

GERTRUD B. UJHELY

Garden City, Long Island, New York
January, 1968

Acknowledgments

This book could not have been written without the prior existence of knowledge about nurse-patient relationships, in particular the conceptual framework developed by Dr. Hildegard E. Peplau. Nor could it have been written if my students in schools of nursing and at workshops in clinical settings had not generously shared their problems and concerns with me.

So many of my friends and colleagues have been kind enough to read, listen to, and comment on selected chapters of the book, or to provide me with reference sources, that I hesitate to list their names for fear that I might forget to mention some of them. My deep thanks go to each and every one.

Special thanks go to Miss Elsa Poslusny who spent a great deal of time in discussing the book with me during the initial stages of planning and who helped me with formulating its outline; to Miss Joan Walsh who read the first draft and made invaluable comments on each chapter; and to Dr. Dorothy W. Smith and the late Dr. Claudia Gips who each read major portions of the final draft and offered comments and suggestions, most of which have been incorporated in the book.

Miss Honora K. Farrell not only listened critically to various drafts of each chapter but also proofread the typed manuscript with me. The encouragement she gave me during periods when the writing progressed slowly was invaluable and is deeply appreciated.

I am indebted to Mrs. Margaret Nolan, Miss Laura and Mrs. Violet Robinson, Mr. Norbert Reuben, and my late sister, Vera, for typing the manuscript from notes that often were barely legible. Finally, my thanks go to Mrs. Helen Behnke for her thorough, careful, and sensitive editing of the manuscript.

G.B.U.

Contents

I

WHAT THE NURSE BRINGS TO THE RELATIONSHIP

Chapter 1

Personal and Professional Values

One of the first things a nurse is taught is to leave personal matters at home and out of the work situation. Why, then, should a book about nurse-patient relationships begin with a discussion of the nurse's personal and professional values?

Of course, it is advisable not to let such personal concerns as one's state of being in love or one's need to defrost the refrigerator interfere with the nurse-patient relationship. Whether this is always possible, even when one's intentions are the best, is another matter.

Values are peculiar in that, unless our attention is drawn to them, we are scarcely aware of having them, much less of the powerful influence they have over judgments we tend to form of people and situations.

What are values? They represent our inner convictions of what is right and wrong, good and bad, desirable and undesirable. They are filters through which we strain our impressions of ourselves and the world around us. They are the bases on which we determine whether to accept or reject an impression, and whether to react favorably or unfavorably to an experience, regardless of whether the experience itself arouses pleasure or displeasure in us. Without values we would not know what to think of the behavior of others, nor how to gear our behavior in response to theirs.

Does that mean, then, that the nurse's relationship with patients will inevitably be colored by her personal values and that advice to leave them out of professional contacts is merely a sign of ignorance? I do not think so. Although there is no doubt that our judgments are determined by our values, we do not have to submit completely to the dictates of those values. We can learn to become familiar with them and to make corrections for them.

To illustrate this point, let us take an analogy from optics. A person who is nearsighted sees the world around him as a general blur, except for very close objects. As a result, the world may appear uninteresting—even unfriendly—to him, for he has no way of seeing its variety, nor can he make predictions about it unless it comes right up to his nose.

If he is not aware of his myopia, he will rely heavily upon his perceptions when formulating judgments. That is, he may easily discount his surroundings as being undifferentiated, dull and uninteresting. He may even consider them as essentially hostile, for they have a way of suddenly forcing themselves upon him when he least expects it. In keeping with his perceptions and judgment, the nearsighted person may respond as follows: He may lose interest in anything that is not directly in front of him; he may belittle it; he may shrink away from it in fear; or he may be ever ready to defend himself against sudden, unexpected apparitions. And, sooner or later, the world around him will probably respond in kind; it may withdraw from him, or it may take advantage of his weakness and throw him off balance.

Now, if this same person is aware of his nearsightedness, several choices are open to him. He can, of course, ignore his awareness and continue to act as just described. But he can also remind himself, again and again, that the only reason the world appears to him as it does is that the lenses of his eyes have a particular curvature, and he can learn to reserve judgment until he has gotten close enough to objects in the environment to focus on them properly. He can also try to reduce his defect through exercises or corrective lenses. If these measures do not improve his ability to see, he can still try to supplement his faulty vision by using his other faculties in addition to his eyes; that is, he can learn to appreciate and even like the complexities of his surroundings by using his ears, brains and hands, in addition to his defective eyes, in formulating his perceptions. This is only an analogy, of course, and has its limitations.

How Her Value System Affects the Nurse's Behavior

Try for a moment, to compare your own value system (the sum of your beliefs of right and wrong, good and bad, beautiful and ugly) with the lenses of your eyes. Just as your lens refracts and focuses your impressions in your own particular way, so does your value system. You cannot get along without some kind of value system any more than you can get along without some kind of lens for adequate focusing. But you can learn to be critical of the impressions conveyed to you by your value system. You can recognize that, although you see things in a certain way, they may appear different to other people. And you can learn to assess the differences by using other media, in addition to your value refraction, when making judgments.

Take, for instance, a patient who is in an advanced stage of Parkinson's disease. He sits there and drools, mumbles something unintelligible if you ask him a question, and spends the day rolling his index finger against his thumb. When he feeds himself, he bends his head over the tray, perhaps with the fingers of his left hand resting on the potatoes, while his right hand spills more of the soup than it gets to his mouth. As you look at him, your value system tells you that such behavior is not appropriate for adults, but only for one- to two-year-old children. Unless you observe your reaction closely, you may find that you are talking to him not as if he were an adult with a neurological affliction but as if he were a toddler. It is only natural for you to give in to this temptation unless you deliberately seek out information about the particular patient's background and about the personalities of people with Parkinson's disease in general, their reactions to their illness, and their feelings about other people's responses to them. Thus, if you ignore your personal values, the chances are that you will automatically treat this patient as if he were a messy child; if you are aware of your values and, in addition, attempt to make corrections for them, you will learn to offer him the kind of relationship to which he, as an adult handicapped by illness, is entitled.

Sources of Values

Early experiences

The values that influence our judgments of others most are usually those we acquired when we were small children. Their adoption was the price we paid for the satisfaction of our early desires. What else could we do? Our needs could not tolerate delay; besides, we were too young then to assess values critically for their worth to us. Remember how you had to share your ice cream with your younger brother if you wanted to have any at all? Or how proud you were when you could lace your shoes all by yourself while your older sister still needed mother's help to do so? No wonder then that today you may still feel strongly about the importance of sharing or of striving for independence. And no wonder then that, unless you check yourself, you may find yourself stating that elderly patients should not be permitted to hoard toilet paper, or that a particular patient who had a cerebrovascular accident is making things hard for everyone concerned because she refuses to help herself.

Cultural and economic background

Let us look at some of the sources of values that are more or less characteristic for certain cultural backgrounds to see how they may affect the nurse-patient relationship unless corrections are made for them. It should be kept in mind that these examples are general statements that may not necessarily apply to every person from a given background. Not only are there great individual differences among members of a group, but there are also different ways of reacting to group pressures. Some people will ingest the values of their environment hook, line and sinker while others may rebel against them and adopt diametrically opposite ones instead. The chances are, however, that every person, regardless of his adopted outlook, retains a certain touchiness when the values of his formative years are contradicted or challenged in any way.

Consider, for instance, the case of a nurse who grew up on the lower East Side of New York. Her father was a tailor whom she hardly ever saw because he worked until late at night so he could afford to send his children to school. She does not remember ever having had a new dress while she lived at home, but only hand-me-downs from older sisters and cousins. Although she and her husband own their own home and have two cars, she often spends considerable time in planning a menu that is based on the current bargains at the supermarket. She is apt to go out of her way to patronize a clothing store that has slightly less expensive merchandise than the one nearby. The fact that she could earn dollars during the time she spends in attempts to save pennies does not enter her mind. This nurse will need to learn that her financial reasoning, although not atypical for people with comparable backgrounds, is not universally valid. Otherwise, she may find herself a harsh judge of a patient who keeps private duty nurses long after there is any medical necessity to do so. She may think of such patients as "spoiled" individuals who pamper themselves more than is good for them. Another nurse, more aware of her own attitude concerning money, may see that same patient as one who, if he must be ill, can at least afford to make himself as comfortable as possible while he is suffering.

On the other hand, consider a nurse who comes from a family where everything goes according to schedule—a family that does not have more children than they can reasonably expect to send to college when the time comes, a family that gives precedence to saving for the future over spending today, that frowns upon eating between meals and that engages in most activities for the sake of their ulterior benefits rather than for immediate gratification. A nurse coming from such a family will have to be careful not to be too judgmental of those patients whose daily stresses of living make the future appear to be nothing but a vague, nebulous unreality. Thus, the nurse who tries to help a mother who has just delivered another baby at home but who has no husband to support it—or any of her previous children—may feel an overwhelming need to teach the mother about the virtue of long-range planning and the necessity for health supervision for all her children. Of course, these are all desirable values, which no doubt would be useful to the mother in the long run. But, at the moment, the woman is harassed by immediate worries. Will the aunt who had promised to come and keep house for her really show up? And, in the near future, will she have to fight it out with the landlord so that he does not cut the heat off too early in the evening, or with the welfare department in order to get enough money to buy second suits of clothes for the older children so they do not have to miss school while their only clothes are drying? She has no objection to health supervision or to starting a savings account, but, in the meantime, she can hardly manage to take one of her children to the doctor when he is really sick, for even then it is hard to get a baby sitter who will mind the others while she spends hours waiting on the clinic bench. How meaningful would the nurse's exhortations be to her at this time? Would they not, in fact, add to the many other unfulfillable demands life is already making on her?

Let us think also of the nurse who comes from a financially comfortable background and whose mother taught her the desirability of being active in organizations that benefit mankind, and of being alert for the newest trends in health and child care practices. It would be only natural for this nurse to consult experts on any area of living, whether the advice she is seeking is concerned with interior decorating, marital difficulties or dental irregularities. But she will need to learn that, desirable as her attitudes may be, they are not necessarily shared by those who would be likely to profit most by them. There is enough evidence to permit us to say that people from lower economic strata, or cultures less sophisticated than ours, tend to get their advice in health matters from family, friends and neighbors rather than from professionals. They tend to seek medical advice for incapacitating, acute conditions but not for long-term illnesses unless they seriously interfere with their occupations. And they will most likely see no connection between self-understanding and an improvement in their lives. Unless the nurse is well aware of deep differences between her value system and those of her clients, she may soon despair at efforts to improve their lots. She may even have to protect herself from facing up to her failure by assuming an attitude of disdain or contempt about these "others" who are "too slothful to participate in human progress."

Ethnic background

An awareness of the values inherent in her own ethnic background may help the nurse a great deal in developing sensitivity to patients from other ethnic groups. Let us take the attitude toward health as an example. If the nurse comes from an "Old American" background, the chances are that she will think of the state of her body in the same way that she thinks of the state of her car. That is, she sees to it that it stays in good running order; she probably has it checked regularly by experts who understand the workings of its surface and various orifices; to keep up its appearance and proper functioning she keeps it clean and oiled; she has badly functioning parts overhauled and will, if necessary (and possible), purchase new parts.

But many patients from less technological societies do not share these values. Although they, too, have theories concerning the maintaining and regaining of health, their analogies are not taken from an industrial frame of reference, but rather from such natural phenomena as heat, cold or the weather. If the nurse wants to be of real help to her patient, she will have to learn to translate her concepts not merely into another language, but also into another frame of reference.

Also, even though the nurse from the "Old American" background is likely to put her greatest trust in the physician who has the most recent training and the most up to date equipment, she will find that some people trust old doctors more than they do younger ones, because they believe that experience counts more than the newest information. She may also find that some patients, particularly Jewish ones, often do not take the word of a single physician but will seek the opinions of two or more experts before they submit themselves to any operation or other major treatment. Other patients are suspicious of the word of any strange doctor unless someone from their own group assures them that he is trustworthy. If the nurse is aware of these differences, she can do much to smooth the way between the physician and his patient, from merely interpreting them to each other to arranging for the kinds of contacts which would make the physician's word acceptable to the patient.

Many nurses do not come from the so-called "Old American" background, but from one of the disadvantaged minority groups. These nurses will have to gain perspective in relation to the double set of values within themselves, for the chances are that, along with the values of their own families, they have also incorporated those of the over-all culture, including its prejudice against the minority group to which they belong. Thus, they may tend to be oversensitive to the behavior of patients of their own group; they may, for instance, expect too much of them when it comes to pain tolerance or patience, as if the patient's behavior reflected on them, too. Or, a nurse may seek out patients of her own ethnic group for special attention, while doing only what is required for other patients, merely because she feels more comfortable with patients who share her cultural background. Other nurses may avoid patients from their own groups so as not to be identified with them, or at least not to give others an opportunity to say that they play favorites. Of course, all of these behaviors on the part of the nurse, although quite understandable, are geared toward meeting her own needs, and have little to do with what may be best for a particular patient.

Although a nurse from a minority group may have risen above any racial or religious prejudices herself, she must be prepared to face the fact that illness often causes a thinning of a person's social façade. Therefore, she is more likely to be confronted with crude hostility about her differentness (whether that be her color, her religion, her language or her body size or weight) by her patient than by the community at large. Fortunate is the nurse who can keep a clear head in these matters and who realizes that even though the patient is entitled to her best professional care, he is not necessarily accomplished in human relationships. And, of course, she does not have to know him socially.

Religious background

Another set of personal values the nurse needs to be aware of is that connected with her religious upbringing. If she is of one of the Protestant faiths, for instance, she is likely to put a great deal of emphasis on the sick person's responsibility for helping in his own rehabilitation. She needs to know that many patients consider their illnesses as acts of fate to which they must submit until destiny changes its mind; these patients are not likely to see any merit in taking individual initiative toward speeding their recovery.

A nurse of Catholic faith may need to be aware of the fact that although close contact with one's spiritual advisor is customary in her religion, this need not be universally so. Such awareness will increase her sensitivity in assessing whether a particular patient should be encouraged to see his minister or not.

Nurses who adhere to the Jewish religion may have to remind themselves that their abstract concept of God and their taboo against two- and three-dimensional representations of Him is unique. This understanding will help them to be tolerant of patients whose religious beliefs lead them to treasure such symbolic articles as the medals they pin to their clothing or the statues they keep on their bedside tables.

Era into which she was born

If the nurse happened to have come into this world around the turn of the century, for instance, she may find it difficult to name aloud certain body parts or functions. On the other hand, a nurse who was born after World War II may find herself in similar discomfort when the theme of death is brought up. Similarly, a nurse who grew up in the depression years may have little sympathy for people who are self-indulgent, whereas a nurse who grew up 15 years later may insist that one make the most of the present moment, since the future probably harbors disaster.

How Personal Values Are Recognized

How can a nurse become aware of these and other values? For one thing, she can try to think back to her early years and remember the kinds of actions for which she was praised and punished. What were the proverbial sayings in her household? What were matters of importance to her parents? Was the past, present or future emphasized most? Which values were stressed more than others—religious ones, intellectual ones, material ones? Was doing more important than thinking, or the other way around? Was work seen as a means for leisure, or as bringing its own reward?

Another way the nurse can find out is to compare notes about her childhood with other people, especially her brothers and sisters, but also friends and older relatives.

Also, she can take notice of the things patients do that seem to bother her most. One nurse may feel very righteous about condemning certain behavior on the part of a patient, whereas another may merely be annoyed by it. Whenever the nurse feels this righteous indignation, she may safely assume that one of her cherished values has been violated—and she can ask herself which one.

A good way to look in on one's values from the outside, as it were, is to read about one's own culture, whether it be fiction or sociological or anthropological literature. The list of suggested readings at the end of this chapter may serve as a starting point for the reader who may be interested in exploring his own value system. Any librarian would be delighted to suggest many additional pertinent sources. Courses in anthropology, sociology, social psychology, philosophy, comparative education and comparative religion are also very helpful. Finally, talking with people from different ethnic or socioeconomic backgrounds or from other countries, and comparing notes with them about customs and do's and don't's, may also help to highlight the characteristic values of one's own background.

Of course, gaining awareness of one's deep-seated values is not something that is accomplished by reading *one* book, taking *one* course or talking *once* with another person. It is a lifelong, ongoing process that needs to be rekindled every time one becomes conscious of having somewhat stronger feelings about a situation than seems warranted by the actual facts.

In time, we can gain sufficient objectivity toward our beliefs concerning right and wrong, good and bad, so as to be able to acknowledge them to ourselves and others without feeling compelled to impose them upon our patients, or to insist that they share them with us.

Values Are Inherent in Professional Practice

Are there some values, however, that in addition to the personal meaning they have for the nurse, also form the foundation of her professional practice? Should she not insist upon adherence to such values as the preservation of life and the promotion of health, and should she not insist that the patient, even though he may not share these values, at least conform to them?

These are difficult and controversial questions for which there is no single answer. On the whole, the nurse can enforce her values in person only with the patient who, for legal or medical reasons, is considered unable to promote his own welfare. For example, under certain circumstances a nurse can force-feed a mental patient in order to preserve his life. To prevent a confused aged patient who is unsteady on his feet from getting hurt, she can sometimes restrict his freedom. But even then the nurse's action needs to be backed by a physician's order.

When the patient is neither legally committed to her care nor in a state of clouded consciousness, the nurse is not allowed to enforce her values, even though the patient may endanger others who are exposed to him physically or emotionally. If the patient's disease is a reportable one such as syphilis or tuberculosis, for example, the nurse can and even must notify the appropriate authorities, but she does not enforce the law herself.

There are also patients who may endanger others but whose condition or action is not legally reportable, such as the office worker with a common cold or the mother who uses "double-bind" communication. In such instances, the nurse can do even less about enforcing her values, even though the office worker may infect his colleagues and even though the mother may cause schizophrenia in her offspring. By virtue of the relationship the nurse has built up with her patients, she can suggest that the office worker stay home or that the schizophrenogenic mother seek psychotherapy, but she can neither enforce her suggestion herself nor cause anyone else to do so. In time, others will take up her point, of course; office workers who lost time because they caught one worker's cold may pressure anyone who dares to expose them to the sniffles to stay home; and once the child exhibits serious pathology, school authorities will probably refer both mother and child for treatment. But by then, much of the damage that the nurse had hoped to prevent is already done.

There are still other patients who seem perfectly responsible and whose condition is in no way contagious or dangerous to others, but who are seemingly bent on destroying themselves. Think of the woman with a breast tumor who does not want to go for a medical examination for fear the verdict may be cancer; or the patient with a lung condition who does not refrain from smoking; or the patient who refuses to have his second leg amputated, even though the operation might save his life. The nurse might try persuasion and point out to the patient that he is not acting in his own best interest nor in that of those close to him. She might also explore with the patient the reasons for his attitude. And she might suggest a joint discussion with his physician or his family. But what if the patient tells her he has given the matter considerable thought and has decided it is best for him and his family not to protract his physical suffering and everyone's emotional agony and economic hardship? And what if he says that life without the pleasures to which he has been accustomed is not worth living? In this case, can the nurse insist on adherence to her value of preserving life at all costs? Legally she has no right to do so. And how about the human point of view? How far can she permit herself to try to influence someone who has made his choice? Is she not burdening him with her attempts to make him change his mind so that he cannot collect himself to face the outcome of his last decision?

I do not think that all nurses will or even can solve this dilemma in the same way. Some nurses may continue to appeal to what is life-affirming in the patient. Others may shrug their shoulders and decide that it is not up to them to alter or question the patient's decision. Some nurses may try to bully the patient into conforming to treatment measures for his own good. Others may try to manipulate the patient by using praise and flattery or even by appealing to their own personal prestige with him.

How the nurse will proceed will depend to a considerable extent on her concept of the patient as a human being or, more accurately, on her concept of human nature in general. That is, does she conceive of the patient as a responsible rational being who must be permitted to make his own decisions, or as someone who is driven by his impulses and must be told by society what is best for him? Does she conceive of his behavior as consisting merely of reactions that have been conditioned by his present state and his environment? Does she see a number of these factors operating?

In Chapter 2 we shall discuss these various viewpoints of human nature and their implications for nursing intervention. Hopefully, this discussion will help the nurse to gain additional insight as to when and why she would, or would not, insist that the patient conform to values held by members of the health professions.

SUGGESTED READINGS

American Nurses' Association. *Code of Ethics*. New York: American Nurses' Association, 1950, revised 1960.

Apple, Dorrian (ed.). *Sociological Studies of Health and Sickness*. New York: McGraw-Hill Book Co., 1960.

Bateson, Gregory *et al.* "Toward a Theory of Schizophrenia," *Behavioral Science, I* (1956), pp. 251-264.

Bell, Norman, and Vogel, Ezra F. (eds.). *A Modern Introduction to the Family*. Glencoe, Ill.: The Free Press, 1960.

Coser, Rose Laub (ed.). *The Family, Its Structure and Functions*. New York: St. Martin's Press, 1964.

Goldschmidt, Walter. *Exploring the Ways of Mankind*. New York: Holt, Reinhart and Winston, 1960.

Gorer, Geoffrey. *American People*. New York: W. W. Norton & Co., 1948.

Hughes, Everett *et al. Twenty Thousand Nurses Tell Their Story*. Philadelphia: J. B. Lippincott Co., 1958.

King, Stanley H. *Perceptions of Illness and Medical Practice*. New York: Russell Sage Foundation, 1962.

Kramer, Judith R., and Leventman, Seymour. *Children of the Gilded Ghetto*. New Haven: Yale University Press, 1961.

Krech, David *et al. The Individual in Society*. New York: McGraw Hill Book Co., 1962.

Lewin, Kurt. *Resolving Social Conflicts*. New York: Harper and Bros., 1948.

Lynes, Russell. *Surfeit of Honey*. New York: Harper and Bros., 1957.

Mead, Margaret, and Metraux, Rhoda (eds.). *Study of Culture at a Distance*. Chicago: University of Chicago Press, 1953.

Myrdal, Gunnar. *American Dilemma* (rev. ed.). New York: Harper and Bros., 1962.

Parsons, Talcott, and Bales, Robert F. *Family, Socialization and Interaction Process*. Glencoe, Ill.: The Free Press, 1955.

Paul, Benjamin D. (ed.). *Health, Culture and Community*. New York: Russell Sage Foundation, 1955.

Riecken, Henry W., and Homans, George. "Psychological Aspects of Social Structure" in *Handbook of Social Psychology*, Gardner Lindzey (ed.). Reading, Mass.: Addison-Wesley Publishing Co., 1954.

Saunders, Lyle. *Cultural Difference and Medical Care*. New York: Russell Sage Foundation, 1954.
Stein, Herman D., and Cloward, R. A. (eds.). *Social Perspectives on Behavior*. Glencoe, Ill.: The Free Press, 1958.
Stein, Maurice (ed.). *Identity and Anxiety*. Glencoe, Ill.: The Free Press, 1960.
Weber, Max. *The Protestant Ethic and the Spirit of Capitalism*. New York: Charles Scribner's Sons, 1948.

Chapter 2

Attitude toward Human Nature

Viewpoints concerning man and his nature can be sorted into four categories: 1) Man is primarily rational and good; 2) man is primarily irrational and bad; 3) man is neither good nor bad intrinsically but merely a product of his environment; and 4) man is a combination of the qualities that characterize the first three categories (1).

These four viewpoints are, of course, very broad categorizations and one can find many variations within each category. Also, no one viewpoint is superior to the others. Each one has been expressed by eminent philosophers and poets and each one has been used as the underlying assumption for the work of great scientists. So, no matter which one of these viewpoints one might recognize as his own, he will find himself in good company.

Our main objective in this chapter is to point out how each philosophy concerning the nature of man can influence the nurse's approach to her patients. We are also interested in the question of whether perhaps one point of view might be more useful than another in certain nurse-patient situations.

Man Is Rational and Good

Let us start with the viewpoint that man is essentially rational and good, a view that implies that man is motivated by kindness and sincerity, that he has respect and tolerance for nature and for other human beings around him. When he is seen as an integral part of nature, nature itself, including the animals in it, is also seen as essentially good. When man is seen as transcending nature, i.e., being beyond and above it, nature may be conceived of as being either good or bad. In either case, however, man is seen as a rational being, able and willing to act humanely in the best interest of himself and others. Should he wander astray through ignorance, he can easily be led back to the right path through logical argument or the good example of others. Should he weaken morally, it would be the result of having been tainted by the evils of corrupt social institutions. (For proponents of this view society is not identical with man; it may well be evil while man is good.) Again, however, an appeal to his inner being will lead man back to his essential goodness. Writers who have expressed this idea include Rousseau, Thoreau, and Emerson. Modern humanists and some psychologists influenced by existential thought also share this outlook on man.

Implications for the nurse-patient relationship

It seems to me that a belief in the basic goodness of man is most useful if the nurse is taking care of a mature human being, i.e., if the patient is a person who has learned to accept himself and the world around him for what they are, or if he is well on his way toward this accomplishment. With such a patient, the nurse is right when she appeals to his reason if, for instance, he neglects to take nourishment because he lacks appetite. With such a patient, the nurse is also right when she applies a little persuasion and even pressure to ask him to do what is best for him in spite of the discomfort this may entail, for she is really only lending reinforcement to what is already highly developed in her patient, and he will be grateful to her for her support.

But let us consider another patient—one who is torn between contradictory impulses without knowing which one, if any, represents his real self. Whenever any impulse gets too strong for him to control, he will give in to it in order to relieve the inner pressure. Then he may be torn by remorse or, if he can't tolerate that either, he may try to justify his act. Examples of such patients are those who overeat, smoke excessively, drink compulsively, and even those who cannot stop themselves from forging checks. If the nurse appeals to the "better nature," will power or reason of such a patient, she is actually adding to his burden instead of being helpful to him. For had he been able to exercise will power, assuming he had some free will to exercise, he would not have gotten into his present difficulty in the first place. And being reminded of his shortcoming is likely to increase his feelings of worthlessness and guilt. Such feelings, in turn, will increase the patient's discomfort and thus push him toward further actions that aim at momentary relief regardless of the future consequences this might entail.

Belief in the primary goodness of man also implies that trust will elicit this goodness in the other person even if it seems hidden for the moment. Such implicit trust can sometimes operate to the patient's disadvantage. Here is an example: A certain patient goes out of his way to please the nurse and do little niceties for her. He shows no sign of sickness and the nurse simply cannot believe that he has committed all the repeated frauds and misdeeds that are listed in his record. If these reports are true at all, she thinks, it is because no one has given him a chance to prove himself. But *she* will be different. She will give him an opportunity to whitewash himself by letting him know that she trusts him and believes in him. As a symbol of her confidence in him, she gives him a key to the ward. And, really, all works out fine; he runs errands for her, keeps himself occupied and useful until, one day, some four weeks later, she is called in on her day off. She is told that the patient has left the hospital without permission, crossed the state line and gotten into difficulty with the law in another state. What will happen between her and the patient when he is brought back? Will she let him know that because of him she almost lost her job? On his return, he will probably find her aloof and unapproachable, for the chances are that he has deeply shaken her belief in the fundamental goodness of humanity. Of course, this kind of behavior is only too familiar to the patient; he has met up with it before—in fact, each time when others made demands on him which were more than he could fulfill. He has become used to being trusted first and rejected later. Why should this nurse have behaved any differently?

Finally, let us consider a patient who had been seriously intent on committing suicide but who now smiles and says he feels much better. The doctors tell the nurse that they believe the patient is dissimulating his depression and that he is more suicidal than ever. They urge the nurse not to let him out of her sight. But this particular nurse feels the doctors are not being fair to the patient. She trusts the patient and cannot believe that he would lie to her. In order to show her faith in him, she relaxes her vigilance, and the patient uses this opportunity to take the only opening he sees to get out of his intolerable agony.

We may state, then, that belief in man's goodness can be to the patient's advantage if he has, on the whole, come to terms with himself and the world around him. But the belief in man's goodness can become a burden to the patient and can lead to serious disadvantages for him if he is unable to live up to the expectations this belief implies.

Man Is Irrational and Bad

Let us look now at the second viewpoint—that man is basically irrational and bad. Among proponents of this belief we find philosophers Hobbes and Schopenhauer, and theologians Calvin and Jonathan Edwards. We find further that much in the psychological theories of Freud and Skinner is based on the assumption that man is basically irrational.

Proponents of this viewpoint see man as nothing but an animal, and they see animals as selfish, immoral beings dominated and driven by instincts, particularly sex, aggression and survival. Hence man must be controlled so that he does not hurt his fellow man. Control is effected by instilling some form of conscience into man. This conscience will then remind him of rewards for good behavior in this or an after life, or it will threaten him with punishment through guilt or the fires of hell. But the moment this artificial conscience is out of action as, for example, after the ingestion of alcohol, or during a massing together of crowds of people, man again experiences an upsurge of the primordial evilness and destructiveness.

Growing organisms need to be selfish

Is there a place for this somewhat pessimistic viewpoint in the nurse's work with patients? I think there is. First (and many readers may disagree with me here), I would say that the selfishness of man is evident in the behavior of children. This does not mean that children must, or should, be deliberately evil and out to hurt others. But by virtue of their being growing and dependent organisms, in order that they may survive at first, their needs have to be met without regard to the needs of others. Thus, without pity, the fetus will deplete the undernourished mother's mineral resources to build his own skeleton. Without regard for the fatigue of his parents or the appropriateness of the hour, the infant demands his food. The two-year-old wants to be loved more than his baby brother regardless of social taboos concerning such egotism. And the adolescent may have to baffle and exhaust his parents through his inconsistent slipping back and forth between independence and childhood.

We must respect this need for selfishness on the part of the child, yet we cannot let ourselves be controlled by it. That is, we must help the mother to protect herself against depletion of her physical resources; we must assess what a baby's nightly vigilance does to the parents' emotional resources and what changes can be made that are not too costly to anyone concerned; we must help the parents to protect the infant from the hostile actions of the dethroned two-year-old, while at the same time providing legitimate outlets for the older child to release his anger; and we must support the harassed parents of the half-grown-ups in enforcing the rules of their household for anyone who lives there, including their rebellious offspring.

Some patients' suffering makes them selfish

The second group of patients who may be described as predominantly selfish are those who suffer from intense physical or emotional pain. Their inner agony threatens to destroy the self and to scatter it into a thousand pieces. To hold themselves together, they must withdraw all available energy from the surface. They are unlikely, therefore, to observe the usual social amenities. Instead, they tend to be uninterested in their surroundings, except for making demands which are often put forth impatiently, without consideration for others. A patient with renal colic is not interested in the fact that the nurse has 20 other patients to take care of who need her too. His pain is threatening to destroy him, and he will probably hold on to the call-bell until the oblivion-bringing needle has pierced his skin. A patient who feels his mounting anxiety tearing him apart, disintegrating him into a nobody, will probably physically clutch the nurse with all his strength. He will not even think of whether she has the time or inclination to stay with him, nor will he worry about the possibility of infecting her with his panic and drowning her in it along with himself.

By asking either one of these patients for considerateness the nurse would be asking him to divert energy from his already weak defense against the onslaught of his pain. On the other hand, she cannot let him pull her down into his agony with him. She would be of little use to him down there. By giving the pain relief at the prescribed time and by reassuring the patient that she will not hold out on it, by staying with him in her strength and not letting him pull her down into his agony, she can support him in his suffering. Her strength will then unite with his forces of self-preservation against the centrifugal pull of his pain.

Some patients cannot tolerate suffering

There is still another group of patients whom one can consider as being irrational and inconsiderate of others. These are the patients who have a particularly low tolerance for any discom-

ALBRIGHT COLLEGE LIBRARY 139026

fort, whether it be an externally imposed discomfort or merely a shift in their own emotions. There is, for instance, the patient who when aroused for his midnight injection thinks nothing of waking the other patients on the ward with his cries of protest. There is also the patient who at the slightest change in routine will become irritable and even belligerent. Finally, there is the patient who wants what he wants when he wants it regardless of whether this is possible at the time. He will get what he wants in spite of the legal or interpersonal difficulties this may entail for him as a consequence or, if he cannot get it, he will throw a tantrum. He may, in fact, under the pressure of this privation, lose his over-all hold on himself and disintegrate as a person.

True, every one of these patients is likely to feel remorseful afterwards. But if a similar occasion were to arise again not one of them would be able to act any differently.

These patients' limitations have to be taken seriously. If possible, such patients should be shielded from sudden shifts in their emotions or at least be prepared for shifts that are unavoidable. Thus, they can be prepared ahead of time for their midnight injections so that they may not have to over-react to their surprise. Similarly, they can be told about anticipated changes in routine and thus be given an opportunity to mentally rehearse the new sequence. With the patient who needs to own the object of his desire, prevention of discomfort is more difficult to achieve. Perhaps he can be encouraged to talk about his need when it arises. Perhaps he can be helped to discharge the—for him—intolerable tension in other ways, i.e., physical activity or diversion to other desirable but obtainable objects. A long bath or shower may reduce his discomfort to tolerable dimensions. But, more often than not, the patient's need will be so great that he is inaccessible to helping influences. All anyone can do then is to keep him physically away from the desired object until the opportunity to secure it is passed. Perhaps in time he can be educated to ask for and apply remedial measures at the first sign of increasing tension. We must remember, however, that this education will be slow and arduous, because the patient's need is overwhelming to him, and all he can think of is quick relief without detour.

Some patients need to vent their aggressiveness

A final group of patients whom one can rightfully consider as being driven by irrational motives and thus as potentially harmful to others, are those whose physical, emotional or social mobility has been restricted for a considerable period of time and who are beginning to mobilize themselves. Some time ago, a French psychologist made a film of children who had been restricted to their beds because of tuberculosis of the bones or joints and who, when they were finally allowed to move about for short periods of time, exhibited a boundless amount of aggression and destructiveness. Many nurses have witnessed the wild frenzy with which a severely depressed or otherwise emotionally immobilized patient may attempt to liberate himself from his inertia. And we are all acquainted with the destruction of human lives and property of which people are capable when they are suddenly freed from long-standing social restrictions.

This seemingly primordial aggression is often incomprehensible to those of us who can discharge our aggression in small doses with every movement, every choice and every statement of self-assertion that we make. Thus, our pent up energy never reaches vast, overwhelming proportions. We would probably not be able to show any better judgment than the people just described if we were deprived—as they are—of periodic opportunities to discharge our aggression. Once the flood is out in the open, there is little we can do except to try to protect the patient and others from serious harm. It is too late to reason with him then.

Perhaps the nurse can forestall such happenings, however, at least with the patient who is under her care. She can assist the physically immobilized patient to get rid of some of his aggression by letting him verbalize his feelings, take part in competitive games and enter into such vicarious experiences as reading detective stories or watching westerns or mystery movies on television.

She can encourage a certain amount of physical discharge in the emotionally immobilized patient through active or passive exercise, or through occupational or recreational projects that are within his grasp, and that involve a certain amount of muscular work. She can reduce some of the pent up emotion by letting the patient linger in a warm bath or shower. And she can indicate to him that she has some inkling of what he is up against in his emotional prison.

Those of us who make home visits to the socially restricted can give them an opportunity to express their hatred verbally and thus perhaps reduce the need for social destructiveness.

We are, then, justified in considering children in general, patients with intense physical or emotional pain, patients with little or no tolerance for discomfort and patients who are restricted in their physical, emotional or social mobility as dominated primarily by irrational motivations and as potentially harmful to themselves and their fellow human beings. We are justified in taking this potential harmfulness seriously. We even have an obligation to apply preventive measures whenever possible and to apply external controls when internal ones prove to be insufficient.

But some of us extend our belief that man is an irrational animal, and essentially bad, to any patient we may encounter. Thus, if we observe that two patients drift toward each other and seek each other out, we may impute that they are governed by purely lustful desires and, as a result, we feel that we must intercede in this friendship. Incidents of this sort happen especially in such long-term settings as nursing homes and chronic disease hospitals where nurses seem to feel a greater responsibility for patients' moral conduct than in short-term settings. But when we separate two such people from each other and strongly suggest that they socialize with all their peers without getting too close to any one, we may be depriving them of a basic human right—the opportunity to develop love and tenderness for a fellow being.

Similarly, we shall have to guard against imputing animal

desires to a patient who reaches out to us physically, even though his gesture seems to be awkward and inappropriate. Often, a physical gesture is the only way he has of expressing to us his feelings of warmth and gratitude. If we frown upon the physical expression of his affection, he may feel that we reject his feelings, and even him as a person, in addition to disapproving of his gesture. It may be a long time before he can permit himself again to feel kindly toward another human being. If we can take his gesture for what it really is, and accept his gratitude and warmth without feeling obliged to return the compliment in kind, we can provide a basis for the patient's learning to express his feelings in ways more compatible with those expected in our culture.

Man Is the Product of His Environment

Now let us look at the third viewpoint concerning the nature of man. People who hold this view believe that man is neither good nor bad, nor even human, until he has undergone a socialization process by other humans. If society around him is good, he will tend to be good too; if society is evil, he too will tend to be evil. Thus, man is merely a product of society. He is, in fact, nothing but the sum total of the social roles he performs. The greater the number of roles he can take on, and the greater the ease with which he can slip from one role into the other, the healthier he is as a person.

The point of view that man is a *tabula rasa*, i.e., a clean slate upon which the environment leaves its imprint, was originally spelled out by Comenius and John Locke in the 17th Century. It is quite prevalent among present-day social and psychological scientists, especially in English-speaking countries. It is the basic assumption underlying the theories of the socialization process as set forth by George Mead and Harry Stack Sullivan. It is the basis of Dewey's theories of education. It serves as a guiding principle for social workers and planners for urban renewal. Nurses' efforts to provide a therapeutic milieu for their patients also bear witness to the importance placed on the influence of environment on human growth.

Helping the patient to know himself

It seems to me that this philosophy is very useful for nurses who work with patients whose self-appraisal has been arrested at a certain level of development. These patients do not see themselves for what they really are. Instead, they still look at themselves with the eyes of earlier, inadequate judges who did not perceive them as persons in their own right but rather as extensions of their (the judges') wishes. Our mental hospitals are filled with such patients, and so are our other health agencies. In order to help these people to grow up and become themselves, we must actually provide them with a corrective social experience which will permit them to re-evaluate their ideas about themselves and in which we take the part of an observer who has no vested interest at stake.

There is good evidence that every human being needs such unbiased observers to help him get to know himself. The human nervous system is so arranged that all our understandings about ourselves must originate from the outside; we cannot directly conceptualize our proprioceptive sensory experiences (2). For instance, if I have a feeling of queasiness or jitteriness—a certain fear of impending doom—I do not know what this means even if I concentrate very strongly on this feeling within me. It is only when I talk to someone else about it (or read about it in a book), and learn that the name of this sensation is anxiety, that I am able to identify it as anxiety the next time I meet up with it. It is also only when I have some understanding of what might cause anxiety (again as learned through others) that I am able to examine my state, to look for its causes, and to search for a remedy for it.

Strengthening the self through strengthening role performance

This viewpoint has another useful implication for the nurse-patient relationship. Since a person's self-view is contingent upon his ability to perform his various social roles adequately, there is a great deal the nurse can do, either directly or through referral to appropriate resource people, to help the person strengthen his role performance. Actually, nurses have been doing this for a very long time, whether or not they have been aware of the philosophical underpinning of their actions. Think of the public health nurse who gives prenatal and postnatal counseling to parents and who helps the new mother with the management of her new responsibilities. Or, think of the psychiatric nurse who talks to the patient, before his discharge from the hospital, about how he plans to handle himself in the light of his relatives' habitual responses to him. Or, think of the nurse in the general hospital outpatient clinic who helps the diabetic patient to reconcile his sick-role with that of worker.

What Constitutes an Ideal Environment

The more help a person can get from his environment in his attempt to understand himself and the responsibilities and skills entailed in his various roles, the more fully he will be able to develop his intellectual and emotional resources. Yet, what today seems to be the optimum kind of environment may be pooh-poohed tomorrow as being highly noxious. Just think of the many different methods that have been advocated for rearing children during the past 60 years. Or think of the efforts in the past quarter of a century to make the hospital a more home-like place for the patient. Recently, there have been some dissenting voices saying that hospitals should represent what they are, i.e., treatment facilities. They should not lure patients into deluding themselves that they have found an ideal substitute home where no demands will be made on them except to go from one scheduled recreational activity to another.

We know very little as yet about what the characteristics of an environment should be that, on one hand, meets enough of the patient's needs to free his energy for growth and recuperation but which, at the same time, by this very meeting of his needs, does not stifle his incentive to unfold himself to full capacity. And we do not know how far we should go in providing shelter for the patient, away from the pressures of the world, where he can be permitted to be as sick as he needs to be without really depriving him, by this very act, from subsequent acceptance in his own community. In fact, we do not even know what groupings are the most beneficial for our patients—those with peers of the same age, those with similar handicaps, or those with people of all ages and all kinds of conditions. It seems that the only way to find these answers is by systematic inquiry. Nurses can and should contribute a great deal to this search.

While skillful manipulation of the environment undoubtedly plays an important part in the growth and recovery of the patient, we need to watch out that the patient does not become a passive pawn in our dealings and that, by his sanctioned helplessness, he does not become an all-powerful monster in his household. By telling the family, for instance, that they must cater to the oddities of the patient recently released from a mental hospital, we are not necessarily helping the patient or his family. Consider, for example, the patient who sleeps all day and stays awake at night listening to the radio. Of course, this may be his reaction to possibly unjustified family pressures, but what does it really do for the patient except to put an unjust burden upon the family who must serve his meals at his convenience and tiptoe during daylight hours, and who find it hard to ignore his nightly noise? When things become too much for them, they are more than likely to throw off the unmanageable burden by returning the patient to the hospital.

Another example is the mother who has hypertension and whose family has been told that even the least excitement could be very damaging to her. Everybody within range of her hearing walks on tiptoe. Her every wish is anticipated before she can voice it. A daughter assumes all chores that used to be her mother's. This woman becomes the passive object of the loving care of her family. But, unfortunately, in our culture a person who has outgrown the stage of early infancy cannot tolerate this passive role for very long. He must reciprocate in some way so as to let himself and others know that he still has some personal autonomy. So the mother tries to hold on to some of the reins in her household but is held back each time by her children's anxious concern. What else can she do but use her power there where it is permissible for her, i.e., in her illness? And, lo and behold, each time one of her offspring wants to take a vacation, or if—heaven forbid—one of them plans to get engaged, she becomes deathly ill. Why not? Are they not trying to leave her, one by one, now that they have made her completely helpless? What would become of her at this point if she were left alone? It would be strange if the children did not resent their mother's exercise of power. But resentment has no place in the relationship with a sick person. It is therefore covered up by increased solicitousness for the patient which, in turn, deprives her more of self-direction and thus calls forth a renewed struggle for power on her part.

It seems then that environmental manipulation is not enough. In fact, it can compound the problems of both the patient and his family. More than this is needed if we want to be of real help to them. Neither the patient nor his family should be viewed as static entities who can be regulated like parts of a machine. Each one of them has inner resources which he can put to work on the problem. We need to help them to bring out these resources and to use them in looking at their mutual bind, to assess it for what it is, and to come up with a dynamic solution which will move the situation forward. To be more concrete, in each situation we can help the participants to examine their behavior and its meaning in relation to the other members of the family. To what behavior of the parents is the sleeping in daytime a response? What is it trying to express in turn? How does it affect the parents? What are the thoughts and feelings of the bedridden patient who has had to abdicate jurisdiction over her household? What does it do to the family to have an invalid in their midst? Neither the family members concerned nor we know the answers to these questions beforehand. But we can serve as catalysts to facilitate communication between them and to aid in bringing about a new synthesis in their relationships. Without siding with anyone, we can ask for each person's thoughts and feelings and for the other's reaction to what was said. We can help them to talk *to* each other rather than *about* each other, and we can help them to explore alternatives which did not seem to exist before. We shall have more to say about these "catalytic" functions of the nurse later on.

Let us recapitulate then the third viewpoint concerning man's nature—that man is nothing but a clean slate subject to the influences of his environment. It is very useful as a basis for providing people with experiences that will correct their self-perceptions and strengthen their abilities to perform their social roles. It can also help to some extent in creating an environment which will foster rather than hinder growth. We need to keep in mind, though, that we know very little as yet about the "ideal environment" for any age or handicap. We also need to keep in mind that we must not, by over-manipulation, lose sight of each person's inner strengths.

Man Is a Synthesis of Good, Evil and Social Influence

Examples of the fourth viewpoint concerning human nature—that man is neither merely good, nor merely evil, nor merely a product of his society, but a combination of all three—can be found in the writings of such great thinkers of the West and East as Plato, Aristotle, Thomas Aquinas, Jaques Maritain, Buddha, Lao Tse, and Suzuki. It also serves as the basis for the work of the psychologists Maslow and Benoit, and of the psychiatrists Horney, Jung, and Reich. The configurations of the three component parts differ with the various writers, but all seem to agree that the main task of man is to achieve a synthesis between the various aspects of his personality rather than mere domination of one over the others.

Three layers of personality

It will have become evident from the earlier discussion in

this chapter that this last viewpoint is also my own. Since a full accounting of the possible configurations among man's good, evil, and socialized self would require more space than this book allows, I shall limit myself to the presentation of one working model which, although somewhat simplified, may be useful to the nurse. This working model leans heavily on Reich's writings, but also draws from other sources (3,4). It sees man's nature as consisting of an outer, a middle, and an inner layer. The outer layer is equal to the socialized part of human nature, the middle one is man's potential evilness, and the inner layer, the core, represents the source of man's essential goodness and his potential. In other words, the outer layer represents that part of man which functions in everyday reality, in close proximity to and in cooperation with other human beings. It is the *persona* (mask) or the *armor* that man puts on in order to perform his various social roles. Most of us are identified with this outer layer. That is, if we are asked who we are, we tend to say we are a nurse, or a mother, or a member of this or that church. In order to keep ourselves identified with our outer layer we have had to ban from our awareness all impulses that might interfere with the various roles we must perform. But banning something from awareness does not really make it disappear. These impulses are collected in our second layer, the layer of potential evilness, the Freudian "id." While all goes well, we are not aware of our middle layer, which is just the way we want it to be. It expresses itself in disguised form only, in our dreams, in harmless competitive games, or in moments of social relaxation, and just enough to release its surplus energy without really harming our outer layer. But sometimes we strive too hard to keep our armor spotless and shining, and we relegate too many of the impulses that are incompatible with it to the middle layer. When the pressure from below becomes too strong, the middle layer is forced into the open by exploding through cracks and weak spots in the armor. At other times it may happen that changes take place on the social stage, or in ourselves, that make the performance of our main roles unnecessary or impossible for a while, or perhaps even forever. Thus, we may find ourselves suddenly divested of our customary outer garment and face to face with our middle layer. That this confrontation is extremely frightening to us goes without saying. We are likely to feel as if a demon had suddenly taken command of our lives. Some of us may submit to this demon and let it act as it wills, while disclaiming any responsibility for it. Others among us may plead for divine or human guidance to conquer this alien force within us and to get rid of it. Again, others among us will try to fight it single-handed, with more or less success. Some of us may let everybody know about our struggles, whereas others may have to withdraw in order not to expose themselves in their weaknesses. We might withdraw from social contacts also in order not to have to be hurtful to our fellow man. Still others among us may try to inactivate the demon, or at least our awareness of it, by magic rituals or soothing potions such as alcohol or an ataractic medicine. Whatever method we use, most of us will try to relegate this middle layer of ourselves to its original place and to forget about it as soon as we possibly can.

Few of us know that because of the way these layers came to be the middle one is, of necessity, also the gateway to the innermost layer. Not until we can accept fully our "evil" and irrational impulses as part of ourselves, without letting ourselves be dominated by them, can we get through to the essence of our being. For the inner layer—that inexhaustible energy pool which is our connection with all of nature, past and present—is the source on which we draw to shape our individual uniqueness and to fulfill ourselves as human beings. It is this inner layer which gives real meaning to our lives, for *it* alone can provide us with a "self" behind the social role. And it is this innermost layer which enables us to transform the activities of the demonic middle layer from sheer destructiveness into new creativeness.

But if few people are aware of this inner core of themselves, even fewer have been able to integrate the three layers of their personalities into their own unique synthesis. These few are the so-called wise men, or the enlightened ones, or—as Maslow calls them—the self-actualized ones (5).

Implications for nurse-patient interaction

The first implication of this three-layer working model for our interactions with patients would seem to be that we must respect the fact that most people are identified with their outer, i.e., their role layers. That is, they conceive of themselves as *being* their various roles. If something goes wrong with an important role, and one has to abandon it temporarily or permanently, he may experience this as a profound threat to himself as a person. It is not up to the nurse to convince her patient that his role represents only one dimension of his total self; if he wishes to penetrate into his deeper layers, he will indicate this in some way. In the meantime, it behooves the nurse to help him in his movement from one main role to another, to support him in the pain which may well be involved in giving up the old and familiar in exchange for the new and unfamiliar, and which often involves irreparable loss, insecurity, and real physical and emotional discomfort to boot.

Support of the patient during role changes. Among the many kinds of role transitions in which we can be of service to the person concerned are the so-called "normal crises" (6), in which a person moves from one stage of development to another: for instance, from preschooler to becoming a school child; from being single to getting married and becoming a parent; from working to retirement; from one geographical and social environment to another as a result of having been promoted to a higher position. We can also be helpful to individuals who experience role transitions that are caused by such "abnormal crises" as the transition from being a child with parents to being an orphan; the transition, temporary or permanent, from health to a sick role or to that of being handicapped; or the transition from being the family's breadwinner in one country to being unemployed somewhere else.

In helping a patient to move from one major role into another, we must be careful not to push him into accepting his present state too quickly. Probably he will have to first go through such various stages of non-acceptance as shock, denial, anger, depression and feeling sorry for himself; all part of taking leave of his old role before he is ready to assume his new role fully (7). If we push for rapid adjustment to his new role, his leave-taking may be slowed up, since part of his available energy may well have to be used to fend off our well-meant admonitions. If, instead, we let the patient know that we have some idea about how his present situation represents considerable change from his previous one, and, if we let him know that we are available to listen to him, should he wish to talk, the chances are good that he will not remain stuck in any one of the leave-taking phases. The chances are also good that he will then take on his new role squarely, whether it be the transitory one of fever-ridden patient, for example, or the more permanent one of in-law.

Sometimes a patient who is about to undergo general anesthesia, or a particularly frightening or painful diagnostic procedure, will indicate to us by his questions that he is afraid of losing his self-control. He may merely ask vague questions, trying to keep us in the room with him, or he may be more specific and ask: "Will I really be unconscious?" "Who will be with me when I wake up?" "Am I likely to say foolish things?" "What if I should start crying or kicking if the pain proves to be too much for me?" These and similar questions should indicate to us that the patient is afraid that his outer role layer (his armor) may not hold up under the massive impending stress and that his second, irrational layer may burst through to the surface.

At such times it would be foolish to encourage the patient to "let go," to "express himself and cry," because this will be "good for him." He has enough to cope with as it is, and should not also have to face this frightening impulse layer if it can be avoided. Rather, we should explain to him the events he is likely to encounter, step by step, so that he does not need to undermine his strength unnecessarily by fearful anticipation of the unknown. We should reassure him that we, or another professional person, will be with him during those moments that are frightening to him, and that we will help him to keep himself in hand. We could also reassure him that if he did say or do anything of which he might disapprove in his waking state, this would occur only in the presence of people who are pledged to hold in strictest confidence anything they see or hear concerning patients.

Being available. Sometimes a patient may say that he feels anxious or uneasy, or that he has certain thoughts or urges that make little sense to him. This is an indication that part of his second layer has seeped into his awareness through a defect in his armor. To help him repair his armor, we can ask him whether there is something concrete that he is uncertain about and on which he would, perhaps, like to get more information. Asking this question will often help him to focus his anxiety on something specific and thus to regain control. The patient may also come up with questions as to how long he will be ill, or how soon will he know the result of his biopsy. If his question has to do with information which we can readily give, I see no reason why we should withhold it. However, if the question has to do with information which only the physician, or someone other than the nurse, is in a position to give, we need to check with the patient first to find out whether he has talked with the appropriate person about it, and take it from there.

Sometimes, however, the patient's anxiety is not merely an indication of temporary insecurity in his role, but evidence of an extensive diffusion of the second layer through the damaged armor. This becomes clear to us when he cannot think of an answer to our question as to whether there is something specific he wants to know or talk about, but continues to complain of his uneasiness or his obsession. In addition to reporting this symptom, we can make ourselves available to the patient should he want to talk more about his discomfort. Without stating at this time whether we think it is good or bad to feel the way he does, we can ask him to describe his feeling to us, to tell us when it started, whether he had ever felt this way before and on what occasions. Of course, we put these questions to him one at a time and wait for what he has to say to each one. This approach will help the patient to regain a certain amount of mastery over his second layer while, at the same time, helping him to integrate that part of it which has come into his awareness and is too large and powerful to be merely pushed back into oblivion.

Protection of the patient and others. We have already talked about the patient who is literally overcome by his impulses and stated that external controls may have to be applied to prevent the patient from harming other people or himself in his desperate attempts to seek relief from his intolerable state. We have also stated that this is not a time when one should try to reason with the patient about the irrationality of his actions; that, in fact, any appeal to his will power might only make him feel more inadequate and would thus further weaken his defense against his impulse. After the episode is over, however, we can suggest that he discuss with us, or another appropriate person he chooses, what happened. Because he has been flooded so extensively by his second layer, he may want to know what it was all about, especially since there is always the possibility of it happening again. If he is acquainted with his second layer, and if he knows the early signs of its impending breakthrough, he may, if nothing else, be able to call for help before it takes over his whole being. There is hope, of course, that gradually he will get to know it so well that he can look at it and feel its pressures without necessarily having to follow its commands.

Many patients will not want to reconstruct what led up to their losing control. They do not wish to be reminded of their terror and humiliation. I think we should respect this need of the patient to forget, even though we may be well aware of the possibility of a recurrence and even though we have an idea that he has gone more than halfway toward his inner core. All we can do in this case is to let the patient know that we, or someone else, will be available, should the time come when he wants to take stock of what occurred.

Occasionally a person may be overcome by a sudden, severe trauma, a prolonged high fever, or an excruciating emotional or physical pain. This experience may be so overwhelming to him that neither role consciousness nor selfish strivings are strong enough to prevent his being swept downstream in it as if in a raging torrent. Unheedingly, he is hurled against rocks and boulders, dropped over giant rapids into churning whirlpools. He perceives himself as a tiny particle without any power of its own. There is no telling whether he will be carried all the way out to sea or whether at any moment he may be thrown against one of the banks where he may be shattered into a thousand minute pieces or where he can regain his foothold, perhaps, and climb out.

Another patient, gradually losing consciousness as a result of sedation, metabolic changes, hemorrhage, or his having given up the fight for life, may feel himself becoming part of the ebb and flow of an infinite benevolent sea around him and may gratefully give himself over to its carrying power, gladly surrendering his individuality to the prospect of everlasting peace.

These are two examples of what it may be like for a person to come in contact with his innermost layer without, however, being able to make conscious use of it at the time for his individual growth. How do we, as nurses, recognize that the patient is in such a state? What nursing measures would be appropriate for dealing with it?

We can get clues concerning the patient's experience from his behavior or from his state: He may show signs of high fever, progressive shock or unconsciousness; he may be apathetic or inert, responding unwillingly to our care or even resisting it with force; he may seem utterly tortured, yet unable to accept, or even to recognize, the help we offer.

Preservation of the patient's individuality. Naturally, we carry out all necessary measures to preserve life as prescribed by the physician. Yet, the way we go about doing this will take the patient's individuality into account, even though for the moment he seems to have relinquished it. That is, even though at this moment he may seem nothing to us but a bundle of weak reflexes, even though he may have forgotten all behavior learned during the early phases of his socialization process, he is still a differentiated human being who may soon again take on his active role in life. We care for his person as he would if he were able to do so. We attend to his skin and mucous membranes, provide nourishment and fluid for him, and we keep his environment fresh and clean. We move him as gently from side to side as if he himself were directing our efforts.

Unless it is medically indicated that we do so, we should not recall him from his inner depth. But we should be ready to receive him when he returns to his surface. The chances are that he will react in one of three ways. He may be terrified of what happened to him, and deny that the realm where he was had anything to do with him as a person by saying that he was "beside himself" or "out of it." Second, he may react to his experience by resenting his return to consciousness and by wishing to go back to that nirvana, where he can again lose himself and forget his frustrations and concerns. A third reaction may be that, perhaps for the first time in his life, the patient begins to realize, in true perspective, the dimensions of his total being. He may be filled with awe of his own depth, the extent of which had not been known to him before. He may look with new eyes at his former strivings: Was it really worth while to have spent all his waking hours in some form of work? Was the pace he kept in doing so really his own individual rhythm, or had he been carried along by the dictates of his times? If these powerful waters that had surrounded him were also his, could he not draw new strength from them each time he felt depleted in his personal resources? He may now recognize the limits of his personal powers and feel smaller than he ever felt before in his adult life. Yet, at the same time, he is likely to feel richer than ever before, having experienced his link with the enormous force of which all living beings are a part.

Whichever of these attitudes the patient should adopt, we will have to respect his choice. Should he have the need to deny any connection between what he had encountered and the way he conceives of himself, we should accept this as a warning sign and not press him toward deeper insight. We may listen to his accounts of the horrors of this "other" world, without trying to explain to him its real nature, for his denial should be read by us as a "stop sign" that the organism is imposing upon itself and others. It says, "You and I may go so far and no further. If you push me beyond this point, I may have to disintegrate."

We also need to guard against judging too harshly the patient who does not wish to return from his state of blissful oblivion. Let him describe his never-never land if he wishes to do so, and as we listen to him, let us refrain from either envy or non-approving disbelief. Rather, let us direct the conversation carefully into the area from which he sought refuge in the blissful state. What are the hurdles in the patient's objective existence that he cannot get over? Perhaps, very slowly, we can guide him into describing what it is that bothers him. Perhaps we can give him, or direct him toward, some concrete assistance in developing the necessary skills to understand and cope with his overwhelming load. It may well be that as he gains skills in mastering his life situation, he will begin to derive pleasure from this exercise of strength and, as a result, the realm of oblivion may lose some of its power of attraction. Frequently, however, the patient who prefers oblivion to his daily life has overwhelming odds against him, in the form of social ostracism, or an accumulation of unsolved problems coupled with a lack of the most rudimentary skills to cope with them. Perhaps all we may be able to do for him while he is under our care is to protect him physically from his efforts to escape, without reprimanding him for what he tried to do. Perhaps all we can hope for during that interval is that our "thereness," our support, will combine with his own strength so that eventually he can begin to venture out to face and remedy his problems.

The patient who has gained a new perspective toward his life is likely to be quite self-sufficient. In fact, we may find him somewhat distant in his behavior toward us, even though polite and pleasant at all times. He may seem very much alone, yet quite content in his aloneness. Perhaps the best way to indicate our appreciation of his experience may be through respectful silence, or perhaps through a symbolic gesture such as placing a freshly picked flower on his tray, drawing open the curtains to let the morning sun stream into his room, or moving the bed to a place where he can look out on the world in solitude.

Should he wish to share his thoughts and feelings with us, we need to be careful in our choice of responses. Timeworn clichés that we so often resort to when we do not know what to say would be very much out of place. Probably no verbal statement on our part could do justice to his experience of inner truth. Our own sensitivity may help us to come up with the right word or gesture that would indicate to him that we have heard and understood.

Summary

In this chapter we have shown how four different viewpoints concerning human nature can affect the nurse-patient relationship. Each has validity in certain nursing situations, but one may be better for interacting with one kind of patient and another for interacting with another kind. Hopefully, our discussion of the last viewpoint has shown that goodness and rationality, badness and irrationality, and the influences of social forces can simultaneously be parts of a human personality. We have also illustrated how clues as to the level or layer of himself on which the patient is functioning at the moment can serve as guidelines for our behavior toward him. If he appears to be identified with his role layer, it behooves us to help him sustain this identification. If his irrational layer has broken through so blatantly that it cannot be ignored, we must protect the patient and others around him from its dangers during the acute stage of this breakthrough. Afterwards, we may suggest to the patient that he become acquainted with his second layer, since it can no longer be ignored. But it is up to him to decide whether he wishes to make use of this suggestion or whether he would rather wipe out the memory of the incident as if it had never taken place. A patient who has to remove himself temporarily from his surface and delve deep into the recesses of his core needs, for that period, our most scrupulous care as replacement for his own. When he re-emerges, we need to observe closely the effect this encounter with his inner depth has had on him. We must also respect the fact that it might either have proved so threatening to him that it cannot be integrated at this time, or that he may have gained a new and total perception of himself with the result that he may have very little need for our advice and counsel. We also need to be alert to the possibility that multiple life difficulties may lead a person into wishing to return to a state of dissolution of himself as a person. We need to do everything in our power to protect him from final harm while he is under our care. And we need to offer, in ways that are tolerable to him, the availability of help that might make it possible for him to learn to carry the load that, so far, has proved too heavy for him.

References

1. Butts, R. Freeman. *Cultural History of Western Education* (2nd ed.). New York: McGraw-Hill Book Co., 1955.
2. Shands, Harley. *Thinking and Psychotherapy.* Boston: Harvard University Press, 1961.
3. Reich, Wilhelm. *Character Analysis* (3rd ed.). New York: Farrar and Strauss, 1949.
4. Jung, Carl. "Two Essays in Analytical Psychology" in *Collected Works, VII.* New York: Pantheon Books, 1964.
5. Maslow, Abraham S. *Toward a Psychology of Being.* Princeton, N. J.: Van Nostrand Co., 1962.
6. Caplan, Gerald. *Principles of Preventive Psychiatry.* New York: Basic Books, 1964.
7. Ujhely, Gertrud B. "Grief and Depression, Implications for Preventive and Therapeutic Nursing Care," *Nursing Forum* 5:2 (1966), pp. 23-35.

Suggested Readings

Benoit, Hubert. *The Supreme Doctrine: Psychological Studies in Zen Thought.* New York: The Viking Press, 1959.

Combs, Arthur W., and Snygg, Donald. *Individual Behavior* (rev. ed.). New York: Harper and Bros., 1959.

Duhl, Leonard J. (ed.). *The Urban Condition.* New York: Basic Books, 1963.

Freeman, Howard E., and Simmons, Ozzie G. *The Mental Patient Comes Home*. New York: John Wiley & Sons, 1963.

Freud, Sigmund G. *Complete Introductory Lectures on Psychoanalysis*. New York: W. W. Norton & Co., 1966.

Harding, M. Esther. *The "I" and the "Not-I."* Princeton, N. J.: Princeton University Press, 1965.

Ingraham, Blanche. "Can the Therapeutic Community be Democratic?" *Perspectives in Psychiatric Care I* (Jan.-Feb., 1963), pp. 31-32.

Newcomb, Theodore M. *et al. Social Psychology*. New York: Holt, Reinhart and Winston, 1965.

Peplau, Hildegard E. "Process and Concept of Learning" in *Some Clinical Approaches to Psychiatric Nursing* (Shirley F. Burd and Margaret A. Marshall, eds.). New York: The Macmillan Co., 1963.

Rapoport, Robert N. *et al. The Community as Doctor: New Perspectives on a Therapeutic Community*. Springfield, Ill.: Charles C Thomas, 1960.

Reich, Wilhelm. *Selected Writings*. New York: Farrar, Strauss and Giroux, 1960.

Rogers, Carl. *On Becoming a Person*. Boston: Houghton Mifflin Co., 1961.

Sarbin, Theodore. "Role Theory" in *Handbook of Social Psychology, I* (Gardner Linzey, ed.). Reading, Mass.: Addison-Wesley Publishing Co., 1954.

Schwartz, Morris, and Shockley, Emmy Lanning. *The Nurse and the Mental Patient*. New York: Russell Sage Foundation, 1956.

Siegel, Nathaniel H. "What is a Therapeutic Community?" *Nursing Outlook 12* (May, 1964), pp. 49-51.

Skinner, B. F. *Walden Two*. New York: The Macmillan Co., 1948.

Stendler, Celia B. "Sixty Years of Child Training Practices" in *Sociological Studies in Health and Disease* (Dorrian Apple, ed.). New York: McGraw-Hill Book Co., 1960.

Sullivan, Harry Stack. *The Interpersonal Theory of Psychiatry*. New York: W. W. Norton & Co., 1953.

Ujhely, Gertrud B. *The Nurse and Her Problem Patients*. New York: Springer Publishing Co., 1963.

Wilmer, Harry A. *Social Psychiatry in Action*. Springfield, Ill.: Charles C Thomas, 1958.

Chapter 3

Educational and Experiential Background

No one doubts that formal education and professional and life experiences influence the way a nurse interacts with her patients. There is disagreement, however, as to whether the direction this influence takes is always really desirable. There is also disagreement as to whether education and experience can produce the same influence and thus are interchangeable.

Some physicians and nurses, too, have expressed concern that nurses may be becoming too well educated. They feel that the nurse, by pushing toward professional status, is really abandoning her unique sister-like role that, in the past, was so important to the patient (1). Some doctors have even exclaimed that they want "hearts" and not "heads" in nurses (2). Some nurses complain that we teach techniques of interpersonal relationships to nursing students instead of seeing to it that they develop kindness in their attitudes and manner (3).

Apparently these critics see kindness and sensitivity on one hand, and the intelligent application of theory on the other, as mutually exclusive propositions. Does knowledge really have to preclude politeness? Does a solid hold on principles really necessitate a frozen heart? Do not all nurses, those with little and those with much more formal knowledge, want primarily to help their patients? Are not both trying to understand what is happening to the patient so that they can do what is best for him at any given time? Is it possible to derive our actions merely from the uniqueness of each patient without having to resort to some form of theory? If by theory we mean an attempt to interpret and explain the phenomena which we encounter, the answer will definitely have to be "No." Except for such reflex actions as withdrawing our hand from a hot utensil, we do not respond directly to the object of a sensory perception, but rather to the image evoked by it in the mind. This image is some sort of generalization arrived at from a composite of previous experiences and learnings concerning occasions resembling the one at hand. And it is this generalization that gives us the meaning of the current situation and shows us the course of action we should take.

Another reason why we cannot simply respond spontaneously to each patient's unique experience but must act on the basis of our interpretations of it instead, has to do with the fact that we have direct access only to our own experience. No matter how close another person may be to us, how well we may know him, and how hard we may try, we can never penetrate the boundaries which separate his individuality from ours. We can never experience his emotions, thoughts or sensations on a firsthand basis. We can only make inferences about his experience from what he says, from the way he appears to us, from what we know about him, and from what we know about our own and other people's reactions to similar situations. The more sources we can draw from to make these inferences and the more trustworthy these sources are, the more accurate our images will be and, as a result, the more appropriate our acts. Thus, if a patient complains of pain in the wound five days after he has undergone an abdominal operation, we have no direct way of gauging the quality and quantity of his pain. We cannot feel it, it is his pain, not ours. However, we can assess his pain by making inferences from what presents itself to us. We can watch his facial expression and his posture. We can listen to what he tells us about the pain. We can recall from the literature and from our experiences with other patients, how much pain he should expect on the fifth postoperative day. We can compare his complaints to those made by other patients we have cared for in the past. If we have gone through a condition similar to his, we can try to recall what we felt like at the time. We can also try to put ourselves in the patient's place by mentally assuming his gestures, expressions and tone of voice. Finally, we can gather all the impressions we have gained concerning the patient's experience and scan our mind for the generalization that would best apply. This generalization will then give us tentative clues as to the kind and origin of the patient's experience and also to possible steps that could lead to its resolution. We may, for example, draw the tentative inference that the patient is suffering from mild, moderate or severe pain; that the pain is probably due to the fact that he has slipped too far down in his bed and is putting strain on his incision; or that it is not the kind of pain normally to be expected on the fifth postoperative day and that some kind of complication must have arisen.

In keeping with our finding, we may decide on one of the following courses of action (which, of course, we shall communicate to the patient): pull him up in bed, or suggest that he do so himself, in order to relieve the pull on the incision; give the routine medication ordered by the physician in the event of pain; or take the patient's temperature and then notify the doctor about the unusual complaint. Whatever action we decide upon, of course, we shall continue to observe the patient closely. Only the outcome of our particular action will tell us whether the generalization we followed was right for the situation at hand. If it was not right, we may have to make more observations and try again for a more suitable answer, or we may have to call in someone who is better equipped than we are to deal with the situation.

Effects of Education on the Nurse-Patient Interaction

Let us examine how differences in nurses' educational and experiential background may affect the inferences they can draw about the patient's experience and, consequently, the way in which they are likely to relate to him. For example, suppose a patient is told by his doctor that he has gastric ulcers and that the most effective form of treatment would be the surgical removal of a large part of his stomach. He spends a few days thinking about this and finally comes to the conclusion that he will submit to the operation, even though he has strong feelings about having the integrity of his body violated and having a part of it removed. He tells the nurse about his decision and asks her to let his doctor know that he wants to see him. In a few minutes, the nurse comes back to give the patient the return message from his doctor—that he expects to see the patient in the early afternoon. But, lo and behold, instead of finding a man resting peacefully after having made his decision, she has a nervous wreck on her hands.

The nurse with little formal knowledge will probably interpret the patient's sudden change of manner in terms of generalizations derived from common sense, that is, he has lost courage, he is afraid, perhaps he does not quite trust his doctor. The element that links these generalizations together is lack of faith in his (and others') ability to overcome the impending threat. The nurse feels that if she can restore his faith, his fear will be lessened and his courage restored. Therefore she proceeds to assure the patient that he has made a wise decision, that his doctor is one of the most competent men in the field and performs this kind of operation every day, and that he should buck up, for all will be well with him in "nothing flat." She means well, of course, and doubtless her patient recognizes this. But, under the barrage of her well-meaning admonitions, how can he tell her that it is his sudden feeling of uneasiness that makes him wonder whether he has made the right decision, and not the other way around?

Another nurse, one with more theoretical background, observes the patient rubbing his hands together, walking up and down in his room, picking up a book here and laying it down there, taking the telephone receiver off the hook and replacing it without having made a call. She associates his behavior with the hesitation and vacillation characteristic of a person who is in conflict, i.e., someone who cannot make up his mind as to which of two (or more) alternatives he should select. Therefore, she decides to give him an opportunity to talk over his conflict with her; perhaps she can help him to resolve it. "Something seems to be bothering you," she says. "If you care to talk about it, perhaps I can be of help?" The patient tells her that he thought he had made the right decision, but now he feels so strange, he is unsure again. He cannot understand why he should feel this way. Thinking that the patient is still in conflict, the nurse attempts to help him explore which two opposing goals might keep him so unsettled. The patient becomes a little irritated. "Look, nurse, I have already thought through all this myself. I have weighed the advantages and disadvantages of operation and no operation against each other, one by one, and I have decided to go through with the operation. So. . .?" The nurse is just as puzzled as the patient. Here is someone who talks as if he were well aware of and able to handle his conflict, yet his behavior belies his words. She tells him that she will report his discomfort and asks him to feel free to call on her if she can be of help in any way. The patient thanks her and resumes his pacing.

Suppose a third nurse were to take care of this same patient, a nurse who has gained some advanced knowledge through formal education or through continued study on her own. The moment the patient tells her about his dilemma, several generalizations come to her mind. She compares each of them to the situation at hand. No, this is not a case of mere preoperative fear, nor is it one of simple conflict. True, the patient *had* been in conflict but he was able to solve it himself and to come to a decision. The phenomenon which she perceives could best be explained by the concept of "cognitive dissonance," which occurs typically *after* one has chosen between two goals, each of which contains aspects of attraction and repulsion. Although the decision has been made in the direction of the goal with the greater number of attractions, one is soon afterwards plagued by the negative aspects of the chosen goal and the positive aspects of the one rejected. Yet, if in light of this experience, one were to reverse one's decision, the same thing would occur again. But once one knows that this is to be expected, one can just ignore the discomfort and put up with it, or one can consciously give support to the positive decision by reminding oneself of additional attractive features it may contain and by finding more unpleasant features for the other. The nurse explains the phenomenon of cognitive dissonance to the patient (without necessarily using the rather awe-inspiring term itself), and asks him whether this phenomenon may perhaps apply to his present predicament. The patient reflects for a moment. Yes, this makes sense to him. It explains to a tee why he would feel the way he does. It assures him also that, under the circumstances, he, or anybody else, would most likely have misgivings after having arrived at a decision. Understanding the source of his uneasiness helps him to tolerate it and to live with it until it subsides. He thanks the nurse for her interest, picks up a book and settles down to read while waiting for the arrival of his doctor.

This example illustrates how additional theoretical knowledge on the nurse's part can be of real help to her patient. Indeed, many nurses feel a serious responsibility to gain knowledge from their own and other fields so that they may better serve their patients. Yet, as they progress through this or that advanced educational program, they begin to realize that no human lifetime would be long enough to master the vast amount of knowledge already available, and being newly formulated every day, that would have relevance for nursing care. No wonder some nurses give up the struggle before they ever try; for what is the use, they feel, they would never be able to gain all the knowledge they ought to have in order to give optimum care to their patients. And they may well say, "A little knowledge can be more dangerous than none."

What is the nurse to do then? She knows that ignorance on her part is to some extent unpardonable because it deprives her patient of the expert care to which he is entitled. On the other hand, in light of what is known and the limits to her time and capacity to absorb this knowledge, she will always be more ignorant than knowing. This is a serious dilemma which many conscientious nurses face in the course of their careers. It is a dilemma shared by people in many other professions and for which no one has yet found an easy answer. For the answer does not lie in merely knowing the key concepts of this or that area of study or in the belief that, if one understands some of its literature and can listen to specialized lectures without getting lost, one has gained mastery of that particular field. Nor does the answer lie in delving deeply into one circumscribed area of knowledge—one psychological theory, for instance—and discounting everything else as not important. So far, no one psychological theory can explain all phenomena we encounter. When we rely too heavily on one kind of explanation we may unwittingly tend to distort the world so that it may better fit our understandings.

Even though there is no general answer to the question, I believe that it is possible for each person to find his own way of solving it. That is, if it is impossible to know all that we perhaps ought to know, let us at least pursue the knowledge that is meaningful to *us* in our own particular way so that we can integrate it well with what we already know and thus can call on it in times of need. This does not preclude our pursuing prescribed courses of study that might help us to become acquainted with knowledge of whose existence we have not even heard. But our personal continued enquiries should follow our own natures. For one person, this may mean an effort to keep up, to his best ability, with what is new, yet well accepted knowledge in his own and allied fields. For someone else, it may mean to pursue further those questions that are raised in his own mind. For a third person, it may mean looking for answers raised by current clinical situations, while for a fourth, it may entail systematic enquiry into a subject that may or may not seem directly related to his work. Still others may combine two or more of these approaches into one.

As we gradually gain more knowledge, however, we must be careful not to delude ourselves that we have reached final mastery of our particular fields, nor should we berate ourselves for past or present imperfections. True, after twenty years of work and study we may shudder at some of the nonsense we committed in good faith in years past. But let us remember that, twenty years from now, we may shudder equally as hard at what now seems to us to be the only right approach. At any given point in our career we will have to act on the basis of the knowledge we have gained so far which, as we know, will always fall short of being absolute. This includes, of course, admitting to ourselves that a situation calls for more knowledge than we can offer at a certain time. Hopefully, in such a case, we can consult with more knowledgeable nurses or professionals from other fields and, if necessary, refer the patient's care to them.

Thus far we have been talking only about the advantage of having theoretical knowledge. There may also be a disadvantage to an intellectual approach that may lend a grain of truth to the assertion that "heads" may be less desirable attributes for nurses than "hearts." We may get so enamoured of the conscious application of theory to practice that we may forget to return from our sphere of generalizations to the unique person of the patient. In other words, we may be tempted to perceive the patient as a case in point for this or that pet theory instead of using the theory as a guide for helping him. We may so delight in the exemplification of what we have learned that we may forget about our reason for embarking on our learning in the first place —the patient and our responsibility toward his care.

Effects of Experience on the Nurse-Patient Interaction

Let us look now at how the nurse's professional and life experiences may affect the way she can interact with patients. Some leaders in nursing are of the opinion that, although professional experience counted a great deal in the past, it is of little significance today. They say, in fact, that years of experience can be replaced, in a much better way, by formal education. It would seem from our discussion up to now that there is some truth in this assertion, for experience, in itself, does not necessarily provide us with the generalizations we may need to solve problematic situations. Does that mean professional experience should be discounted altogether? Does it mean that a nurse barely out of school can be as effective with her patient as another nurse who has practiced for many years and who has lived a life rich in joys and sorrows? I do not think so.

First, the more experienced nurse can make authoritative statements derived from her past observations that would sound presumptuous if made by a novice. Take, for instance, a patient in labor. She indicates that she has come to the end of her endurance, that she cannot take one more minute of what seems an eternity of suffering ahead of her. The experienced nurse can assure the patient that in this particular stage of labor many other women have felt as she does at this moment, and yet it is a sign that things will come quickly to a head. This statement, coming from a nurse who looks and acts as if she really has helped hundreds of women have their babies, will ring true to the patient and may well give her the strength she needs to again participate actively in her arduous task. A similar reassurance given her by the novice nurse may well have the opposite effect. "How would she know? I may well be the first woman she has seen in such pain!" And what was meant to be supportive by the nurse may instead heighten the patient's loneliness and feeling of despair.

Here is another example: A patient with a schizophrenic reaction complains of a feeling of inner strangeness, of "not being herself." She keeps asking the nurse what may be causing this feeling. The new practitioner acts correctly if she asks the patient to describe her discomfort, if she asks her to tell her more about when it started and under what circumstances it gets worse. The young nurse is right also if she asks the patient to defer the question of causation until they both know more about the facts involved than they do now. But this is as far as she can go, I think, without overstepping her bounds. The experienced nurse, even though she does not have the answer either (for who does, except the patient herself, eventually), can offer some additional reassurance to the bewildered patient. That is, on the basis of having observed many patients in similar distress, this nurse can authoritatively say that this feeling of not being herself is part of her illness, that it is likely to get worse if she concentrates on it, and that as she gets better, it will gradually disappear.

The experienced nurse, backed up by what she has encountered in the past, may also give *advice* to the patient. She can suggest that the patient make an effort during their time together (or with her therapist) to explore what has led up to her illness, but that at other times she should try not to brood about her state but rather participate in the various available activities even though they may not seem to grant her much relief. She can *predict* for the patient that this (even though it does not show at once) will help her find the cause of her condition much more quickly than continually focusing her attention on her state. Similar advice given by a novice nurse may easily be interpreted by the patient as presumptuous or as a sign of ignorance.

The experienced nurse can also assess better than her younger peer when a patient should be encouraged to try harder and under what circumstances she should let him be. For example, after having made one round of his room on crutches, a patient shows a certain amount of strain and fatigue and expresses the wish to rest for a while. The experienced nurse can tell whether she should urge him to continue a little longer in spite of what he says, or whether she had better go along with his request. How does she know? She does not really know in advance, any more than does her junior colleague, exactly how much effort she can safely expect any given patient to put forth. However, she is able to compare the minute nuances of his tone of voice, his bearing and expression with those of many others she has cared for, and this will give her subtle clues as to his capacities. The new nurse, still without this reservoir of guiding hunches, will have to take the patient's word for fact, since misuse of persuasion may well overtax his resources, or it may increase his reluctance to go on. In other words, the new practitioner, in spite of perhaps equally good grounding in theory, will—for the patient's safety—have to be much more conservative than her more experienced colleague. That is, she will have to take a slower route to obtain desired results.

Yet, there may also be advantages in being a new practitioner and disadvantages in being an experienced one. To the novice nurse (except perhaps while she learns to recognize various diseases) each patient is a live person whose predicament presents a new, awesome and immediate reality for her. The seasoned nurse, however, will have to guard herself from viewing the patient in his condition as merely another example of something she has seen many times before. She may have to remind herself that what can have become a routine event for her, is anything but routine for the patient, and that it is easier to observe than to be the main participant.

Having had personal experience with events similar to those that trouble patients can, of course, also be most valuable for the nurse. She can project herself into the patient's situation if she, too, has given birth to a child, undergone an operation, or suffered the loss of a loved one or a part of her body, and has learned to accept this loss.

On the other hand, we must guard against expecting that the patient will interpret his condition in the same way as we did ours. Each event that befalls a person is interpreted by him in light of his past experiences and his present knowledge, and his interpretation of it will color his experience of it and the way he responds to it. Having had a successful cancer operation may mean for us that it payed off to go for our yearly checkups. It may mean that we were fortunate the condition was found in time and that we need to be alert to any symptoms which might indicate a recurrence but that, on the whole, we can gratefully expect to resume our lives where we left off. To a patient, on the other hand, the word cancer may mean ultimate doom and disintegration. His operation may have been just as successful as was ours, yet in light of his interpretation, he may prepare himself for early death instead of being grateful for renewed life. It is important then that, although we may have had a condition similar to the patient's, we be alert to what it means to him and do not take his interpretation of it for granted in light of what it meant to us.

The chances are that each one of us will have to help patients with experiences which we have not undergone ourselves, for not all of us have delivered babies, and few among us have undergone psychotic breaks. Only a minority of nurses have personally experienced brain or heart surgery, and although some of us have been close to death, none have actually crossed its threshold. We cannot hope, then, ever to have first-hand information of all conditions for which we are asked to be of help. Perhaps it is better this way. It helps to remind us, again and again, that each living being is an entity to himself, essentially alone, who must cope with his problems and his sufferings in his own particular way. And it is just because we are separate from the patient, just because we are not also in the midst of his predicament, that we can be of real help to him. Our energies are not bound up in his struggle. They are free and can be used to assess his difficulty in its proper perspective and to look for possible ways out of it. They can be used to lend support to the patient so that he can lean on them and free some of his own strength. Our energies can also be used to clear somewhat the path that he can or will have to take, and to walk along beside him, step by step, at his rate and as far as he (or we) can go.

References

1. Caplan, Gerald. *Concepts of Mental Health and Consultation; Their Application in Public Health and Social Work*. Washington, D. C.: U. S. Department of Health, Education and Welfare, 1959, p. 265.
2. Vaillot, Sister Madeleine Clemence. *Commitment to Nursing*. Philadelphia: J. B. Lippincott Co., 1962.
3. Wolff, Ilse S. "The Educated Heart," *Amer. J. Nursing* 63:4, (April, 1963), pp. 58-60.

Suggested Readings

Allers, Rudolf. *Existentialism and Psychiatry*. Springfield, Ill.: Charles C Thomas, 1961.

Brehm, Jack W., and Cohen, Arthur R. *Explorations in Cognitive Dissonance*. New York: John Wiley & Sons, 1962.

Buber, Martin. *I and Thou* (2nd ed.). New York: Charles Scribner's Sons, 1958.

Campbell, Norman. *What is Science?* New York: Dover Publications, 1952.

Festinger, Leon. *A Theory of Cognitive Dissonance*. Stanford, Calif.: Stanford University Press, 1957.

Hillman, James. *Suicide and the Soul*. New York: Harper and Row, 1964.

Hughes, Everett. *Men and Their Work*. Glencoe, Ill.: The Free Press, 1958.

Lewin, Kurt. *Dynamic Theory of Personality*. New York: McGraw-Hill Book Co., 1945.

Lewin, Kurt. *Field Theory in Social Science*. New York: Harper and Bros., 1951.

May, Rollo. *Existential Psychology*. New York: Random House, 1961.

Peplau, Hildegard E. "Process and Concept of Learning" in *Some Clinical Approaches to Psychiatric Nursing* (Shirley F. Burd and Margaret A. Marshall, eds.). New York: The Macmillan Co., 1963.

Shands, Harley. *Thinking and Psychotherapy*. Boston: Harvard University Press, 1961.

Tillich, Paul. *The Eternal Now*. New York: Charles Scribner's Sons, 1963.

Ujhely, Gertrud B. *The Nurse and Her Problem Patients*. New York: Springer Publishing Co., 1963.

Chapter 4

Physical and Emotional States

Desirable as it is that nurses be in an optimal state of body and mind during their working hours, this cannot always be achieved. The nurse is as prone to headache, malaise, fatigue, apprehension and anger as the next person. Yet, being a professional worker, she needs to be aware of the effect any one of these conditions may have on her relationships with patients.

How the Nurse's Physical State Affects Her Interaction with Patients

Some nurses disregard any discomfort they may be having while they are at work, but in ignoring their discomfort they also tend to ignore that part of themselves that is involved with it.

Malfunctioning sense organs

Consider, for instance, the nurse whose eustachian tubes have become somewhat blocked following a common cold. Although her cold has subsided, she has a constant humming sound in her head, an uncomfortable feeling of pressure, and she also does not hear well. Until she sees her doctor again she cannot do much to relieve her condition except to take the prescribed drops and pills. So she is back at work, with her doctor's consent. She tries to put her trouble out of her mind during duty hours. But, together with her discomfort, she ignores the difficulty she has with her hearing and, before she realizes it, she becomes irritated with a patient because he does not speak loudly enough for her to hear. Since she has never before complained to this patient about his low voice, and since he feels he is speaking to her as loudly as he always has, he may easily conjecture that she is displeased with him or that she is picking on him for no good reason. Had she acknowledged her difficulty and told him that her ears were giving her a bit of trouble, and had she asked him to raise his voice so she could hear him better, he would gladly have obliged.

It is important then for the nurse to remain aware of any handicap in her functioning that may be associated with physical discomfort, and to admit it to the patient if necessary, in order to forestall misunderstanding and hurt feelings on his part. There is no need, of course, to burden the patient with a lengthy case history as to the cause, duration and possible outcome of the condition.

Slowed reactions

Sometimes, for example, under certain weather conditions, or when our acid-base balance is slightly off, or when we have not had a restful night, we have the sensation of being behind a thick wall of fluff. With some effort, we can get ourselves to talk but our voice sounds muffled, as if it came from far away. We try to reach the other person, but the wall imprisons us. We strain against it, try to penetrate it and shake it off, without success. We become irritable; if we cannot get out ourselves, why does no one lend a hand to take the wall away? Things become worse when patients start making demands on us. We find it hard to fulfill them because it is difficult to move fast enough. The more demands we receive, the more we seem to slow down. It seems to us that just because we do not feel right today, the patients are asking more of us than is their custom and are less willing to wait their turn. It may be true that they are irritable and demanding. It may be that they, too, are affected by whatever has imprisoned us; or perhaps they are merely offended by the fact that we do not quite meet their expectations. Yet, irritability on the part of either of us will not get us closer to each other. It might help, though, if we were to remark—in a matter-of-fact way—about the atmosphere (if that seems to be the cause), or about our state. Perhaps the patient feels the same way we do. In this case, he may be relieved to find out that what he feared was a relapse is merely a not unusual response to atmospheric pressure. But even if he is not as "cobwebby" as we are, we can ask his indulgence for our slowness until we can free ourselves from whatever it is that is holding us back. Admitting our state to ourselves and to others, instead of vainly struggling against it, will very likely lessen its effect on us and gradually, we will be able to remobilize ourselves and get back into our usual swing.

Pain

Sometimes the nurse will be in pain due to some transient disturbance such as dysmenorrhea, headache or a gastrointestinal upset. If possible, she should alleviate this pain before she comes into contact with her patients, for it is very hard to concentrate on the suffering of other people while one is having pain onself. The nurse needs to be alert to the fact, however, that as she obtains relief from her discomfort, the contrast between the sensations, or perhaps the medication itself, may create a sense of well-being in her that is not in keeping with her usual nature. She needs to watch this feeling of expansiveness for it may cause her to be less perceptive and less careful than she ought to be. It may even carry her into rash decisions that are based on her own state of being rather than on what the patient needs.

Fatigue

Sometimes, when spending many hours with just one patient, especially at night or right after having eaten, the nurse may become drowsy. When she notices that her eyes are getting heavy and her attention is wandering, she should not just stay put and pretend that she is wide awake, because the patient who expects her to devote her unflinching attention to his care may feel insulted if she sits there and nods as he addresses her. She cannot help feeling sleepy, of course, but she remains responsible for what she does about it. She is entitled to, and should therefore feel free to, request relief for as long as it might take her to splash cold water on her face, take a breath of fresh air, or even leave the ward to have a cup of tea or coffee.

How the Nurse's Emotional State Affects Her Interactions with Patients

Anxiety

On occasion, the nurse will experience considerable anxiety, because of matters at home that may concern her, or because of circumstances at work. She may find that she asks twice for each direction and that she forgets to do many of the things she is supposed to do. She finds it hard to grasp the meaning of her patient's message, except in its strictly literal sense. She finds it impossible to organize her day, since she can see only its parts, and not the way they fit together.

Here again it is important that the nurse acknowledge her state of being to herself. If it is at all possible to do so, she should postpone direct contact with patients while her anxiety level is high, because she may infect them with her apprehension and thus increase theirs (which may already be present in too large amounts). Thus, the patient's anxiety level may be increased to such heights that, in some cases, it may trigger a state of panic.

Even though the nurse may not be able to do much about the reasons for her uneasiness at the moment, she can do something about controlling it. Activities which require physical exertion or repetitious actions such as making empty beds, straightening out instruments, medicine bottles or Kardex notes, are some effective ways of reducing one's anxiety to manageable size. There are many such chores in the nurse's work area that may have long waited for the appropriate moment to be done.

Of course, the nurse will have to let her peers know that she is trying to get herself back in hand by keeping herself occupied with these tasks right now, and that she will soon resume her direct care of patients. Let us hope that her colleagues will understand and respect this need and will not, by their displeasure, make things more difficult for her.

Sometimes, even though she is upset, the nurse has to remain with the patient. In this case, she will have to try to do the best she can within the limitations set for her by her anxiety. That is, she cannot hope to make valid inferences or connections between past, present and future events. She will have to put up with a field of perception that has narrowed and which, because it can focus on small details only, is not able to survey the whole situation. And so, in caring for the patient, she will proceed very slowly, deliberately checking each step for error or omissions. And in spite of the fact that her thoughts tend to scatter in all directions, she will give herself concrete, concise orders that will help her to keep focused on her task. Any drawing of conclusions, interpreting and teaching will have to wait until she can think comprehensively again. If something must be taken care of right that moment, she will have to ask someone else to assist her.

Should the patient note her inner unrest and question her about it, it would be only fair to him that she admit to the difficulty. Denial could lead him to doubt his own powers of perception, or to wonder what it is about him that is so distressing to his nurse. There is no need, of course, to discuss with him the reason for her apprehension, except to make sure to let him know that it has nothing to do with him.

Anger

The nurse may also be very angry at times. Members of her family or her co-workers may have irritated her. She may be furious because the day off for which she had made special plans was changed at the last minute, and she was not even asked whether she would mind. Or she may fume in exasperation about the social system at her place of work that bucks every effort she makes to initiate improvements. Sometimes she will be able to get rid of her anger by expressing it directly to the persons concerned, or by integrating it into the remainder of the painful experiences she has learned to take in stride. At other times, however, she will still be filled with annoyance when she is about to give patient care. Then she will need to inform her patients that she knows she appears to be ready to pick a fight, but that it is not they who have made her angry. She may even ask them to try not to test the limits of her patience until she is able to gain control over her explosive state. This would spare them looking for what they might have done to arouse her disfavor. It would also increase their respect for the nurse as an alive human being who is able to experience a wide range of emotions and who can acknowledge them without, however, needing to let them loose on the first victim who crosses her path.

It would not do, of course, to discuss the reasons for her anger, or any other private emotions she might feel, with the patient. He may have to learn that professional workers are human, too. Acceptance of this fact may even help him to become more realistic in his expectations of the nurse. But it would violate the ethics and even the nature of a professional relationship if the client were asked to focus on the helper's troubles instead of being aided in resolving his own.

Effects of Ignoring Physical or Emotional Unwellness

If it should happen that the nurse is seriously unwell with an emotional or physical disorder, she should not (as many nurses think they must) drag her sick self to work. Not only might she expose her patients to her illness but, while being ill herself, she is in no state to be of help to them; she needs all her energies for meeting the demands of her own system. Any outside request must, therefore, represent an added strain for her, which may reduce even further her capacity to be of help. Also, it is when she is not well that she may slip up and make mistakes in giving medications; it is then that patients and staff may find her being curt, irritable and sometimes downright rude to them. At the slightest provocation she may lose her temper altogether, because one tends to resent those to whom one gives more than one has to offer, even though one may not be consciously aware of one's resentment at the time.

Afterwards she will be sorry, of course, and may ask herself how she could possibly have lost control like that. Apologizing and stating that she was ill may not improve the matter, since the others may seriously wonder what kind of nurse would take on the task of helping others before she has learned to help herself.

Yet, many a nurse feels that she must go to work regardless of her physical or emotional state. She may be in dire need of money, and may not have any sick-time pay coming to her. Or she may feel that she cannot let her colleagues or her patients down, especially in situations where there simply is no one to be found who could possibly take her place. This is a serious dilemma that the conscientious nurse faces. If she needs to work because she cannot afford to lose her pay, she will have to decide for herself where the greater danger to her security lies—in losing one day's pay or in running the risk of being fired because she is more likely to make mistakes, perform below par or get into interpersonal difficulties with patients, families or staff. She may also have to consider whether her need for money outweighs the risks she imposes on those who are forced to come into contact with her illness. Besides, she may have to consider what more lasting damage and subsequent loss of pay may be created by overtaxing her body at a time when it needs all the rest it can possibly obtain.

As to the nurse's fear of imposing on her colleagues by increasing their already too heavy load, one may wonder whether a period when the nurse herself is incapacitated is really the best time to attempt to solve the staffing problems at her place of work. Perhaps these should have been looked at by her, together with her peers and superiors, while she was well and could have contributed fully toward their solution? Reporting for work when she is ill may, in fact, only perpetuate the situation. Of course, we all know that numerous institutions in this country and abroad are run, day in and day out, by a skeleton staff. One person's absence naturally creates a major disaster. There is no doubt that this problem is urgently in need of solution. If only they were asked or would dare to speak up, staff nurses might have valuable suggestions for reaching this goal. They might, for instance, do as some other professionals are doing and make some of their own time available to pools from which help can be drawn in case of staffing shortages. More importantly, they might help to examine what is wrong with nursing service in the first place that it does not attract the necessary quota of nurse practitioners to fill its needs. Is it low salaries? Poor personnel policies? Lack of an inservice program? Does it have to do with the attitudes which filter down to the ward level from the top? Does it have to do with poor communication, lack of recourse for grievances, or perhaps all of the above named things? Since not all institutions suffer from a nursing shortage, there must be some explanation of why some do and others do not.

Of course, we all know that in institutions that operate year in and year out on an emergency basis, or in which conditions are conducive to job dissatisfaction, nurses are more prone to take time out to be ill. On some occasions, the nurse's physical or emotional state may be such that she *could* go to work, but what adds weight to her decision to stay is her aversion to having to face another day of harassment from the head nurse, supervisor or the auxiliary workers assigned to her; another day of not being permitted to contribute what she really has to give; another day of having to "run herself ragged" because there is no one else to help with the work. Under any one, or a combination, of such circumstances it is understandable that the nurse may take the easy way out. If, however, she sees herself repeatedly leaning in this direction, she needs to take the initiative and do something about the situation. If she can do this, fine; if she cannot (this she will only know if she leaves no avenue for change unexplored), she should consider seriously whether her present place of employment is the best one in which to exercise her talents.

Some nurses, particularly those employed in psychiatric settings, feel that they must go to work, even when ill, for they have promised their patients they would be there and a professional person must never break a promise. How realistic is this outlook? What if the nurse were dead? What if she were held captive in her home by a band of burglars? Could she stick to her promise then? "Well, no," she may answer, but these would be circumstances far beyond her control. But what about illness? Perhaps she might have been able to prevent her condition had she been more careful in managing her over-all resources; perhaps not. Once she is actually ill, however, is this not also a circumstance beyond her control which needs to be taken as such and respected? "Of course," the nurse may say, "but my patient needs me. And as long as I can get to his bedside, even if I have to crawl, I must not permit myself to let him down. For the first time in his life he has developed some faith in another human being; he trusts and believes in me. Just think what it might do to him if I were to break my promise and let him down."

Well, he might be terribly disappointed. He might also be very angry with his nurse. And, for a while, he might even retreat into his old, suspicious self. In the long run, though, would he not be better off coming to grips with the fact that he has begun to trust this nurse even though she is not really a superhuman creature? Actually, she never did pretend to him that she was all-powerful. In fact, she had told him at the outset that she expected to be there whenever she said she would, except if anything were to interfere over which she had no power, and then someone would notify him as soon as possible to that effect. And she had kept her promise. She came every time she had said she would, except once when she was held up by a flat tire; even then she called and left a message that she was delayed, and that she would be with him later. Sure he was upset then, too. But what more could she have done than she did do in effect? This time, too, he was notified that she was ill and that as soon as she herself knew when she would be back she would leave word for him as to the date. What more can he expect of her? Perhaps he was right to trust her after all. More importantly, he may feel that if there is one human being who, although not infallible, is worthy of his trust, who knows, he might some day meet others like her.

Suggested Readings

Manaser, Janice, and Werner, Anita. *Instruments for Study of Nurse-Patient Interaction*. New York: The Macmillan Co., 1964.

Peplau, Hildegard E. "A Working Definition of Anxiety" in *Some Clinical Approaches to Psychiatric Nursing* (Shirley F. Burd and Margaret A. Marshall, eds.). New York: The Macmillan Co., 1963.

Chapter 5

Attitude Toward Her Professional Role

Many people, including nurses, have an aversion to the use of the term *role* in connection with human relationships. It has for them the implication of acting, of playing a part, instead of being oneself, and thus connotes phoniness and insincerity.

There is a certain amount of validity to this objection that is based partly on the intrinsic meaning of the word itself and partly on the phenomenon which we described in Chapter 3, i.e., that most people are so identified with their various roles that they do not differentiate between self and role. They see themselves as being their roles rather than assuming them.

Definition of the Term "Role"

The term "role" was, in fact, originally used in the theatre (1) to denote the rolls on which actor's parts were written. Later it came to mean the part itself. Gradually, although the term retained its theatrical meaning, its use was expanded to include the part a person plays in a real life event as, for instance, Jefferson's role in formulating the constitution of the United States (2). Finally, the term role came to mean also the behavior assigned to and expected of a person in a certain social position (3).

There is truth also in the fact that one feels most comfortable with oneself when one fulfills one's assigned roles (such as the sex role or the role of son or daughter) and one's chosen roles (such as that of teacher or choir member) in the expected way. Those who deviate too far from a culturally prescribed range are likely to experience personal guilt, whether or not they admit it to themselves.

In societies that are less complex and more stable than our own, role and self are practically one and the same. One is cast into his role at birth—a role clearly outlined by virtue of one's father's caste, class and occupation and also by one's sex. Thus, one has no choice but to be one's role. The Victorian housewife, as prescribed by her role, was truly a chaste, weak female who leaned on her husband for economic and muscular support. In return, she supervised the household and the nurturing of her children. She also submitted to her husband's sexual wishes, but was not permitted to admit that she had any of her own. Any deviation from this role would have been most shocking to her contemporaries. It would have been a sign that she was "not herself."

Complementarity of Roles

Carrying out one's roles involves more, however, than just one's own behavior. Roles have a particularity of interlocking, of being reciprocal. That is, the role of one person, since it is not enacted in a vacuum but in relationship with others, predetermines to some extent the roles of others with whom one interacts. Thus, for the Victorian couple, the fact that the wife enacts the role of a weak woman who leans on her husband with all the weight of her helpless, fragile frame automatically casts her spouse into the complementary role of protector and provider. We need not be concerned in this instance as to which role causes which complementarity. We do need to remember, though, that one role will call forth complementary role behavior in others. Further, we need to remember that changes in one person's role will cause some changes in the roles of all those with whom his role interlocks.

What happens when one's roles become more in number and at the same time more ambiguous? Think of today's suburban housewife about whom so much has been written lately (4, 5). She is her husband's wife, mistress, companion and housekeeper; her children's mother, chauffeur, teacher, friend and party hostess; her neighbor's competitor in more ways than one; her club's secretary; her friend's counselor; and what not. Her interpretation of her over-all role might be very different from what her husband expects it to be, depending on each one's ethnic, financial and geographic background and the values that would go along with these. Also, the expectations society may have of a person in her position are likely to alter periodically in accordance with her husband's advancement in his job, particularly if this also entails changes in their way of life and residence.

Yet frequently, neither husband nor wife are exactly clear as to what the role change implies, except that it should be in accordance with social expectations. Because our society is oriented to the future, we feel that we must not turn to our parents, or to tradition, to find clear-cut guidelines for ourselves. Instead, we turn to our contemporaries who, for the same reasons, are also unsure of themselves. And so, each one watches the other for clues as to the appropriateness of his actions, but these clues, like the husband's job promotion or his salary increases, come as *responses* to their actions rather than forewarnings. No wonder then that people tend to be rather tentative about the manner in which they dare enact their roles toward each other, their children or the world at large. They cannot afford to present a clear-cut image which may be the wrong one as far as the others are concerned, for this may lead to their being disapproved of, ridiculed or, worst of all, being rejected and thus relegated to isolation from their peers.

Since there is an interdependence between role and self, a blurred image of one's social roles results in a blurring of the outlines of one's personal identity. If one is not sure of *who* one is, one cannot very well trust one's own judgment. It is only natural, therefore, that one turns to others to find out how well one has performed one's role. Yet, turning to others, unless they are unbiased observers who let one's self be as it is and help it grow, cannot strengthen one's feeling of identity; on the contrary, it will weaken still further the discriminatory powers of the self.

How Role Perception Affects the Nurse's Interactions with Patients

Now, what does all this have to do with nursing? I think it has a great deal to do with it because the nurse has her fair share of problems related to her perception of her role and ways of enacting it clearly toward others in light of the many changes that have taken place in nursing.

Mothering—the nurses' historic role

In the past, her role was primarily a mothering one (or, in some countries, that of an older sister). Her main task was to nurture and provide comfort for her patients. Hence, her activities centered around bathing the patient and caring for his body, providing nourishment for him and feeding him; changing his bed linen and airing his room; reading to him; wheeling him out into the sun; and so forth. In recent times, the scope of the mother's own role has been enlarged considerably, but many people, including members of the nursing profession, expect nurses to continue to function within the confines of the mothering role of the past. Now, there is nothing wrong with the mothering role per se. In fact, it is the one most indicated in the nursing care of acutely ill patients, small children and very dependent adults. But modern nursing comprises many other areas of activity in which mothering per se would not be appropriate—in problem solving, for example, or prenatal counseling for responsible adults, or the administration of complicated procedures, or the carrying out of research.

The modern nurse has many roles

The idea that the role of the nurse is a mothering one is so widespread, however, that many future practitioners still expect to be prepared primarily in the nurturing aspects of patient care. Yet, as they progress through the educational programs they have chosen, they begin to see that nursing comprises many roles in addition to the traditional one of mothering; in order to graduate, they will have to demonstrate some proficiency in the technical, managerial, teaching, socializing and counseling roles as well. In fact, since students are less likely to be familiar with the subject matter comprising these other roles, more emphasis may be placed on their mastery and less on the mothering role. This practice, however, unless the reasons for it are made very clear, may easily lead to misunderstandings on the part of students and young graduates. It may give them the impression that their earlier expectations were merely signs of ignorance and that the mothering role does not really belong in the repertory of full-fledged nurses. No wonder, therefore, that once they graduate, they may feel that it is perfectly proper to refer all tasks and activities connected with mothering to auxiliary helpers.

Teacher and counselor. Certain roles are used so frequently in certain clinical specialties that they seem almost characteristic for the specialty itself. Thus, one often associates the teaching role with public health nursing and, lately, the counseling role with nursing in psychiatry. It is because certain clinical areas provide such rich opportunity for the practice of certain roles that they are selected by preservice educators to introduce the student to the role as well as to the clinical content itself. Thus, the technical role of the nurse is often emphasized in connection with medical-surgical nursing and her teaching role is emphasized in connection with prenatal care. Focus on the counseling role may be delayed until the student reaches the field of psychiatry, sometimes not until her last year. Although concentrating on one role in each specialty may make it easier for the student to learn the content of that specialty, it may also create misconceptions. Unless the contrary view is clearly pointed out to her, she may easily come to believe that, in each field of study, only the role stressed by the teacher is important and that the other roles have no relevance and can simply be ignored. And so, when they get out of school and into practice, they may, for instance, tend to disregard the physical symptoms of psychiatric patients and neglect reporting them or according them the proper care. Yet, psychiatric patients can communicate less well than others what troubles them and they are often less willing to submit themselves to physical aspects of care. Would it not, therefore, behoove a nurse working in psychiatry to be doubly alert to untoward physical signs in her patients? And should she not be especially skillful and deft with her fingers in order not to overtax their already low tolerance for being touched?

Physician's assistant. Nurse practitioners who work in an emergency service may focus exclusively on the task of assisting the doctor as he reduces a fracture or puts stitches into a wound. They cooperate with him splendidly and anticipate his every move. He does not have to ask for a single instrument, sponge or special medication. This kind of role performance on the nurse's part is, of course, highly praiseworthy. It enhances the speed and safety of the procedure and thus helps a great deal in preventing unnecessary physical suffering for the patient. But while she concentrates on facilitating the doctor's work, could she not also have one glance or one word for the patient? Obviously not. To her, surgical nursing is synonymous with technical expertise and nothing else. Whatever she may have learned concerning reassurance by helping to reduce the patient's fears, has been filed away with the information concerning other clinical specialties for which she has very little use now that she has graduated and chosen her own field.

Each role has its place in the patient's care plan

Because each role is taught to them as an entity, some nurses, although able to move from one role to another in a given situation, find it very difficult to enact more than one role at the same time. This difficulty is illustrated by the story of the proverbial student who gave her patient his bath, arranged his bed and his room and made him as comfortable as she knew how, without speaking a single word to him. When she was finished, she asked him whether he was comfortable. He said he was; whereupon, she pulled a chair to his bedside, sat down facing him and said, "Very good, now that your physical needs are met, I shall try to meet your emotional ones."

This may appear to be ridiculous behavior, yet the student showed some wisdom in what she did. It is helpful for the patient to know which role or roles one is about to assume so that he knows what is expected of him. This way, he can assume a role complementary to ours without unnecessary groping about and thus squandering his much-needed energy. Hence, a private duty nurse who is caring for a patient suffering from a long-term illness may well make plans with him as to how she will distribute the time she devotes to carrying out her several roles. She may, for instance, reserve an hour in the morning for her counseling role when both she and the patient can take a look at the impact his illness has had on his life. They can also, perhaps, try to recall important events prior to his illness which may have played a part in leading up to it. And they will, hopefully, establish ways in which he can plan to cope with things in spite of and within the confines of his condition.

She will reserve certain times during the day for discharging the technical, mothering and managerial aspects of her role. She will give him fresh drinking water, bring him his tray and keep him company while he has his meals. She will bathe him, massage his body, help him with prescribed exercises and take care of dressings that need to be changed. Of course, should the patient talk at these times, she will listen skillfully and help him to enlarge on the topic on which he has embarked. But it is not necessary for her to expect, or even to encourage, that he focus on himself during the entire day. Quite the contrary. In fact, she will plan for times in which her socializing role will be predominant; for instance, she will help him to keep up-to-date on current affairs to the extent that he can concentrate on them without showing fatigue. She will also encourage him to keep up his outside contacts by helping him with phone calls or with letters. As the occasion arises, she may do incidental teaching while she gives him care, but she will set aside times when he is most alert and rested to concentrate on such subject matter as procedures he will have to learn before he goes out on his own, or how he can select menus he likes within the confines of his special diet. This way, the patient can organize himself accordingly and does not need to "tense up" in anticipation and fear of what she might be up to next each time she leaves and enters his room.

Most nurses, however, are not able to spend an entire day with one patient. Especially if they are experienced in their work, they may have to combine a counseling session, or the discussion of current best-selling books, with administering a bath. And they may have to start teaching a patient how to perform a procedure simultaneously with doing it themselves. However this combining of roles may not always be feasible for new practitioners. A young nurse, for instance, who is trying hard to find the urinary meatus of her patient in order to catheterize her, may not be able to concentrate at the same time on the patient's voicing her fear that perhaps she will never again be able to urinate normally. In this case, the nurse has the right to tell the patient that she will discuss this topic with her after she has completed the catheterization, but she must also be sure to make time for listening to the patient as soon after the procedure as she possibly can.

Even when the nurse is assigned to one patient, it is not usually possible to spend an entire day on one role, except perhaps the mothering and technical one with someone who is critically ill. For instance, a counseling session is hard work both for the patient and the nurse. It requires a great deal of concentration and self-discipline for the patient to look seriously at himself and for the nurse to listen to what the patient says he sees and to guide his looking. Keeping this up for many hours might well exhaust them both. Besides, new insights need time to evolve slowly, without continuous prodding from the outside; they also need time, once they are out in the open, to align themselves and be integrated with other aspects of one's self. Nevertheless, students are sometimes required to maintain their counseling role with one patient for an entire day. Other students, especially those in psychiatric settings, may be used almost exclusively for socializing with patients. One wonders how many hours one not specializing in recreation can profitably spend in playing gin rummy or chinese checkers. It is not surprising that both students and patients lose interest after a while. Although continuing with their game as they were told to do, they may well detach themselves internally from one another and each pursue their private fantasies.

Differences in the Ways Nurses Evaluate Their Roles

They give precedence to the role they like best

Some nurses become so enamored of one of the roles they have learned that they will try to apply it at all costs, whether or not the patient's condition warrants its use at the time. Thus, some nurses feel the urge to set up a counseling session with any patient they encounter, regardless of the circumstances surrounding their meeting. It is true that the nurse needs to be available, or tuned in at least, to listen for cues from patients that they wish to confide in her. But she does not need to grasp every opportunity of their being together to provoke such confidence on the patient's part. This might well meet her need to be his advisor, but what will focusing on his psychic troubles do for the patient who, on his way to the x-ray department, has slipped halfway off the stretcher and is in urgent need of being lifted back onto it?

Other nurses may be so intent on their role as teacher that they will proceed without stopping to see whether the anxiety level of the patient whose health habits they would like to improve is low enough to make it possible for him to learn, or even to hear what they are saying.

They use their roles as status symbols

For certain nurses, some roles seem to carry more prestige than others. Thus, a nurse may go around the ward and talk with her patients whenever she has some free time. However, if one of them should ask that his bedpan be removed, she would not dream of doing this herself, but would call on an aide instead.

Another nurse may have become imbued with self-importance following her promotion to the I.V. team. It is, indeed, awe-inspiring to watch her deftly draw several syringes of blood from the patient's vein and inject it into tubes and bottles without spilling one drop on his spread or her immaculate white dress. Her manner toward the patient is so aloof that, when she is through, he does not dare ask her to raise the head-end of his bed and pull his breakfast tray closer. Besides, it would be too late —she has already left the room.

Still another nurse may feel she has "arrived" if she can spend all day in the nurses' station, answering the telephone and writing out medicine cards, laboratory slips and x-ray requests. If a patient should come to her door with a question, she is likely to brush him off with "Please, don't disturb me now, can't you see that I am busy?" Of course, patients will be impressed and intimidated. But will they also have confidence that these nurses will be available to them in times of need and that they will do the right thing at the right moment? I doubt it.

They adapt their roles to patients' needs

Fortunately, there are many nurses whose actions are guided by the patient's state and the over-all requirements for his care rather than by their own predilections for certain roles. Patients appreciate being skillfully lifted on and off bedpans just as much as they appreciate being listened to; they appreciate a warm breakfast as well as having unbruised veins; they appreciate receiving a medication soon after the doctor orders it. They also like to think that their questions are welcomed.

Difficulties Nurses Encounter in Carrying out Their Roles

Adverse working conditions

Often the setting in which the nurse works makes the judicious application of her various roles impossible. Suppose she is the only nurse assigned to evening duty on a ward with 30 very ill patients. She has no choice but to try to carry out all those procedures that must be performed by a registered nurse. This leaves her with practically no time for fulfilling any other role and forces her to delegate all other aspects of care to her aides. Even so, she is lucky if she can complete the required procedures before the night nurse arrives. Of course, she knows that some patients harbor all kinds of fears and would benefit from having her spend some time with them, but she has barely enough time to instruct the aides about what to do. She is already late in giving pain-relieving medication to three patients who have requested it and need it badly, but that cannot be helped either, since the intravenous fluids of several others are running low and have to be replenished. Also, she can no longer delay taking the vital signs of two critically ill patients.

Working under such circumstances must be very difficult for the nurse who would like to put into practice what she has learned. Why doesn't she quit and find work somewhere else? Why should she? This is already her third position. The first two had been in settings that were exactly like this one. Why doesn't she go back to the good clinical situation where she received her basic education? Well, she feels that was an artificial setting, arranged especially for teaching purposes—not the real thing. Is the setting she is in now real? Obviously. All the other nurses say it is, too. What about all she had previously learned about the roles of the nurse? Well, that was just theory. Teachers believe in it, but nobody who has to give actual service can cling to these ideals and survive. One has to do the best one can. One has to continue living with oneself. And so she continues, day in, day out, trying to do at least the things that are most essential, looking forward to her days off and contemplating going to school in order to get out of the "rat race."

In the meantime, what has happened to her relationship with patients? Well, she is pleasant enough and tries hard to do the best she can for them. She has little genuine warmth, however, little sincere interest in them. She cannot afford to be interested because she cannot really follow through on what this would imply.

What does working under such circumstances do for her identity as a nurse? Very little, I fear, since she does not really enact the roles that would strengthen her identity and make it apparent to herself and others. What she represents, to herself and to them, is the image of a workhorse rather than of a professional nurse. Of course, workhorses will be used as such—that is what they are for. A workhorse also rarely decides whether his work is suitable for him; this is for his master to decide. In the case of the nurse, the master may be the supervisor, the admissions office, the administrator, doctor or the patient. They make the assignments and she carries them out to the degree that she can, that is, up to the limits of her strength.

This is a rather bleak picture. Exaggerated? Not really. We all know that today nurses have to give a much greater number of medications than they formerly did and carry out many complicated procedures which the physician used to do. We also know that the shortage of professional nurses is critical in many institutions. Does that mean, then, that there is nothing the nurse can do about it? No. There is a great deal the nurse can and will have to do about it. For it is *her* identity as nurse and, consequently, also as person, that is in question. Her potential for giving the kind of care her patients are entitled to goes along with this identity. Therefore, she cannot really submit passively to conditions as they are, nor can she wait for others to alter them, although it won't be easy to do otherwise; it will take both courage and strength. She will have to find, within herself, a faith in her own identity, and strengthen it since the faith she once had has been lost through external circumstances. That is, she will have to keep in mind and develop trust in the main focus or concern of her profession. She will have to learn to believe in this core concern, in spite of demands and pressures from all those who feel entitled to her services, because keeping centered on her professional focus will best aid her in learning how to state the conditions under which she will accept employment. It will also be her guideline as to how many and which of the proposed tasks she can take on and still retain her identity.

Clarity of Role

A clear image of the nurse's professional identity

If she is really convinced of her identity and of what her profession has to offer, she will also get this image clearly across to others. Her boundaries will no longer be hazy and she will no longer act as a vacuum into which others are drawn to expand their own roles but, instead, her outline will be clearly defined, not merely by words, but also by actions which speak for themselves. She will, for instance, state how many patients she can take care of. She will request the supervisor to assign an additional nurse to help with the work she cannot manage to do alone. She will not be afraid to stand up for what she thinks is necessary in the interest of her patients. If she has the quiet courage of her convictions, her superiors may very well go along with her. They may even find that other nurse to help her even though this seemed out of the question at first. After a while, they may note comments made by patients about the excellent care they have received. And who knows, they may in turn put pressure on the administrator to take a better look at staffing patterns and to modify them so as to give nurses an opportunity to nurse.

Adherence to the central core of nursing

Since roles have a way of being reciprocal, it is possible that a consequence of the changes that occur in nursing may be that other professions will, in turn, have to make adjustments in their own boundaries. That should not be too serious a problem, though, for other professions seem not to have lost their identity as nursing seems to have done. Even if they have to adjust their roles to some extent in order to better articulate with ours, it would not necessitate a basic reorganization on their part. Further, once we believe more strongly in our identity and the core-concern of our profession, we need not be afraid to adjust our roles to accommodate changes which may well occur in theirs in response to changing needs, for, by that time, we shall be able to talk and negotiate with others in light of our own identity instead of merely tending to follow the directions we receive.

References

1. English, Horace, and English, Ava Champney. *A Comprehensive Dictionary of Psychological and Psychoanalytical Terms.* New York: Longmans, Green and Co., 1958.
2. *Ibid.*
3. *Ibid.*
4. Spectorsky, Auguste C. *The Exurbanites.* Philadelphia: J. B. Lippincott Co., 1955.
5. Friedan, Betty. *The Feminine Mystique.* New York: W. W. Norton & Co., 1963.

Suggested Readings

American Nurses' Association. *ANA in Review* 13:2 (1965).

Benne, K., and Bennis, W. "What Is Real Nursing: Role Confusion and Conflict in Nursing," *Canadian Nurse* 57 (Feb., 1961), pp. 122 ff.

Hartog, Jan de. *The Hospital.* New York: Atheneum, 1964.

Kluckhohn, Florence, and Strodtbeck, Fred L. *Variations in Value Orientations.* Evanston, Ill.: Row Peterson, 1961.

Krech, David *et al. The Individual in Society.* New York: McGraw-Hill Book Co., 1962, Ch. 14.

Meyer, Genevieve Roggy. *Tenderness and Technique.* Los Angeles: U.C.L.A. Institute of Industrial Relations, 1960.

Newcomb, Theodore M. *et al. Social Psychology.* New York: Holt, Reinhart and Winston, 1965.

Peplau, Hildegard E. "Principles of Psychiatric Nursing" in *American Handbook of Psychiatry* (Silvano Arieti, ed.), *II* (1959).

Riesman, David *et al. The Lonely Crowd*. New Haven, Conn.: Yale University Press, 1950.

Smelser, Neil J., and Smelser, W. T. *Personality and Social Systems*. New York: John Wiley & Sons, 1963.

Vaillot, Sister Madeleine Clemence. *Commitment to Nursing*. Philadelphia: J. B. Lippincott Co., 1962.

II

THE CONTEXT WITHIN WHICH THE RELATIONSHIP TAKES PLACE

Chapter 6

The Nursing Profession

Although nurses talk a great deal about roles and about the tasks and activities relevant to these roles, there is no concensus about the central idea that binds all these roles and activities together. Yet, what else but a central, underlying theme could give our roles, tasks and activities their reasons for existence? What else could support our defense of them as being at the core of our work?

What is this core concern of nursing that will help us to maintain our sense of self? Do we know what it is? Are we even aware of it? Have we had it in the past but lost it? Was there ever such a thing? Nurses give rather vague answers when asked these questions.

The Focus of the Profession Determines the Practitioner's Actions

It is this special focus or "core concern" of his profession that outlines the practitioner's field of action and helps him to select from all available knowledge and skills those that are most useful for his purpose. His specific focus also determines the stage, or over-all framework, for his relationship with his client, other professionals, and the community at large.

The focus of a profession need not remain the same throughout the ages. Some professions were not even in existence one hundred, or fifty, or even twenty years ago. Others have either shifted their focuses or expanded their core concerns in light of the emergence of new knowledge and changes in cultural patterns. Thus, medicine used to be (and still is in some societies) a function of the priesthood. In Western society the two callings have gradually become separated, although some missionaries of our time still practice both of them. In earlier times, physicians were more interested in classifying and treating diseases than in preventing them, because very little was known about disease causation. Since the advent of Pasteur, Koch and Freud, however, much biological and psychological insight has been gained concerning the etiological factors which can produce disease. This has resulted in a widening of the focus of medicine so that it now includes the area of prevention as well as those of diagnosis and cure.

On the other hand, advances in technology and science need not necessarily lead a profession to widen its *focus*; it may merely call for an extension of its *tasks* and *activities*. Thus, new instruments and new techniques have widened the field of surgery considerably and have made treatment and cure available to many more people than one might have dreamed possible not too long ago. Yet, all these innovations in medical practice have left the core concern of medicine undisturbed.

The client has some idea of the central concern of each profession, even though he may not have actually seen it defined in print. Thus, if he is reasonably well informed, and if he is in a position to make a choice, he will seek out that professional who, because of his particular preparation, is most likely to be able to solve his problem, or what the client believes to be his problem at the time.

As the various health professions have enlarged their scope of practice, a certain overlap in activities has occurred. This has led to power struggles in certain settings, and has also led some professionals to raise questions as to their true identity. Yet, need a father question his identity, just because he helps his wife with the dishes and occasionally changes the diapers of his son? Not unless he tries to determine his identity on the basis of what he does. It is doubly important, therefore, that one's professional identity be established by the core concern of one's profession, rather than by taking stock of one's activities.

Since the nurse-patient relationship is a direct outcome of the way nurses view the core concern of their profession, it behooves us to look into what nursing considers to be its central focus.

The Core Concern of Nursing

All authors agree that the main concern of nursing is, or should be, the patient. Some even say that it is the whole patient that nursing should be concerned with—the patient in all his dimensions—physical, emotional, social and spiritual. Then, after having said this, authors seem to get sidetracked into describing either what they think nursing is or should be, the main functions of the nurse, or what the tasks and activities are which characterize the profession.

Thus, for instance, in the early part of this century, the nurse was seen mainly as the physician's assistant—an extension of him, as it were—who, by her persuasion, induced the patient to use his will to live and get better (1).

Since that time, however, much has changed. Only a few of the nurse's functions are still dependent functions (2). Hence, the focus of today's nursing goes beyond being merely an extension of the physician's role.

Nursing is a kind of teaching

Annie Goodrich, at the outset of collegiate education for nurses, saw that one of the nurse's chief concerns is her role as a teacher (3). She was right, of course; teaching is an important part of nursing. Yet, we know that there are many nurse-patient situations in which, because of the patient's condition, the teaching role does not apply.

Nursing provides comfort

More recently, the nurse has been seen chiefly as a provider of comfort for the patient (4). It is true that this is her principal function in many cases and probably should be true in many more. Yet, does not the nurse have to hurt the patient occasionally in order to be of real help to him? Does she not have to insist that he breathe deeply after an abdominal operation, even though this may cause him to have more pain? Does she not have to change his position often in spite of the discomfort this may entail for him? In order to help him face and cope with the realities of his life, the nurse must sometimes hold up the truth to him or must ask him painful questions. Often the nurse cannot afford to keep the patient comfortable, for this would result in keeping him ill or aggravating his present condition.

Nursing provides an optimal environment for the patient

For a long time, the nurse has been seen as that person who provides an optimal environment for the patient (5,6). Lately, especially in the field of psychiatry, this idea has been extended to include the emotional climate on the ward (7). In fact, this responsibility is often seen as the exclusive concern and role of nursing. Is this where nursing has its beginning and its end? I do not think so.

Because of the increasing complexity of hospital services, some authors feel that the nurse should function primarily as a coordinator of all aspects of the patient's care. Others disagree, saying that the essence of nursing is direct practice at the patient's bedside—not administration from a central desk.

Many of today's nursing leaders agree that the nurse *cares* for patients. This is a good term, for she administers care to the patient and she cares what happens to him. Yet, the term is not specific enough, in itself, to be the kernel around which the nurse can develop her professional knowledge and the tasks and activities derived from it.

Nursing involves caring for the whole patient

Some authors are more specific (or, more inclusive, perhaps). They say that the nurse cares for the *whole* patient, that she gives him *total* nursing care by meeting all his needs. I wonder, however, whether this is possible in the majority of nursing situations? No one can meet the total needs of another for any length of time. Of course a mother meets all of her baby's needs during its intrauterine existence and the first weeks of its life outside the uterus. The nurse, too, in her mothering role, renders total care to patients who are in critical condition, unconscious, or too young to be able to dispense with being mothered. She not only meets but also anticipates their needs. But are there not many patients whose needs we could not possibly meet, even if we tried? Some have serious financial and interpersonal needs; they are in debt and they are lonely. They may also be in need of clothing, sexual satisfaction, or a job. True, we can aid these patients in assessing their needs and in getting the help they require for meeting at least some of them. It is doubtful, though, whether we can really meet all these needs ourselves.

Some patients do not want total care from us in the first place. All they want, and perhaps all they need, from us is instruction about how to manage their colostomies and all the paraphernalia that go with caring for them. If we tried to find out how they are getting along at work and with their families, or whether having the colostomy may have kept them from attending church regularly, these patients might well think we were imposing on their privacy. They may be proud. They may want only what they think they *need* from us, and no more. They may not want our "total" care, at least not at this time.

Nursing is a helping relationship

Several writers (8, 9) have defined nursing as a helping relationship. Although it is true that nursing is a helping relationship, would not the practitioners in other professions also want to think of their relationships to their client as helping ones? "Helping," like "caring," is an attractive term; but does it carry enough specificity to describe what is unique to nursing?

Nursing helps patients to learn from their experiences

Other writers see nursing as a professional relationship in which the patient and the nurse are helped to profit and learn from his experience of illness (10, 11, 12). This may be a most gratifying relationship for both nurse and patient, for sometimes the nurse can be instrumental in helping the patient reach the stated goal. Yet, very frequently indeed, patients merely want to feel better. They do not wish to learn from their experiences; in fact, they wish to be permitted to repeat the same blunders as often as they feel like it, without being reprimanded or censured. Some patients simply do not have the strength for deeper understanding of themselves or of their current situations. Of course, we need to be available to the patient to help him integrate his experience and learn from it. But I do not think that we can expect every patient to want or even to be able to accept our offered help.

Nursing has not yet been defined

Some writers state that we do not know what nursing is and that we must define it before we can decide on what constitutes nursing practice. Others, while basically agreeing with this statement, claim that the definition of nursing is intimately connected with what we know about man himself. The more we know about man, the better we shall know what nursing is or should be (13). This is an important argument that cannot be just laid aside. On the other hand, man needs care now. He cannot wait until we know everything there is to be known about him. Besides, a great deal is known about man already and there is no limit to what still needs to be found out. Suppose, however, that we had all the facts about man at our fingertips; would this really tell us more about nursing? Do we not need a central focus around which to organize this knowledge so that it will be meaningful for us? This reasoning brings us right back to where we started: What is this central kernel from which the meaning and the uniqueness of nursing—and all the know-how that goes with it—can be derived?

In its Position Paper on Education (14), the American Nurses' Association has attempted to synthesize these divergent viewpoints by stating that the "essential components of professional nursing are care, cure and coordination." Each of these components is seen as encompassing a broad range of activities and judgments on the part of the nurse.

Nevertheless, the questions, "What is nursing?" and "What is unique in nursing?" continue to plague members of the profession at their faculty meetings, and wherever nurses congregate to talk about their education and practice. Apparently, all nurses feel the need to find the hub of our independent nursing functions—the focal point which would make it possible for us to determine what comprises the unique body of knowledge belonging to nursing, and to define the proper scope of nursing activities.

Lack of clarity of our professional focus is, of course, evident in the actual practice of nurse practitioners and in the questions they raise about the purpose of their relationships with patients. Yes, they can see that time could profitably be spent with a patient in order to elicit his life history or to find out about the genesis and early symptomatology of his present condition. They have learned the importance of this from the physician with whom they work and who often directs them to obtain such information for him. Of course, they would also like to comfort the patient, to take his troubles away, if they only knew how. Yet, the more they allow him to open up to them, the more they are aware of the fact that his problems are larger than they and he can deal with, and that the only result would be that they too would be burdened with these problems.

It is no wonder, therefore, that some nurses refer the patient to other professionals as soon as he begins to open up about himself, that others avoid any kinds of discussions that might leave them helpless and stranded, and that others merely restrict themselves to giving physical care—teaching, perhaps, or exhortation. If they turn to their teachers or supervisors for help, they are frequently not much better off, for these people, too, are either caught up in the profession's dilemma or they offer a somewhat one-sided approach which may or may not be applicable to the actual situation.

Sustaining the Patient Is the Real Concern of Nursing

In the discussion which follows, I shall propose one possible way in which the central focus of the nurse-patient relationship might be viewed, and which could possibly get us out of our deadlock. I am, of course, aware of the fact that this need not be the only or the best solution.

A long time ago, Florence Nightingale stated that "nursing . . . is to put the patient in the best condition for nature to act upon him" (15). Perhaps we would do well to retain this idea and merely rephrase it somewhat in keeping with our present enlarged scope of health practices. Today's patient (or client, as many non-medical workers call him) needs help not only to overcome his illness but also for handling such matters as making the best of his personality; finding a place for himself in a new community; being a good parent to his children; and living within the confines of his handicap. Today's patient (or client) is in desperate need of someone whose expertise consists of *sustaining him in his experience* of struggle, whether it be the crisis of a serious accident or emergency operation; childbirth or the death of a close relative; having to live with a face badly scarred by burns; having to live with one's tendency to project one's shortcomings onto others; relearning to speak after a cerebral accident; or facing death after repeated heart attacks or in the last stages of leukemia. Who can better fill this need than the nurse? Who but the nurse often stays round-the-clock with the patient, is frequently present during various interventions of other professionals, and is able to interpret the patient to the other professional and the professional to him? I would certainly not disagree with those who may believe that it is the clergy's duty to sustain the patient, but not all patients avail themselves of religious guidance, nor is the clergy likely to be present throughout all the critical moments of the patient's illness. Besides, as we have already mentioned, there may very well be an overlap in the activities of various professional groups. And so, although ministers of various denominations certainly play an important role in sustaining people in their life experiences, their main concern, or so it seems to me, has to do with helping to bring God closer to their parishioners and vice versa. This chief concern of the clergy may also be one of the concerns of the nurse who is sensitive to her patient's spiritual needs, whether she does or does not belong to a religious order. Her main focus, however, has to do with *sustaining the patient through the experience* which has brought him into contact with her in the first place. As for nursing today, the phrase "sustaining the patient through his experience" should probably not be qualified by such words as "health and disease" or "convalescence." The health-illness dichotomy is not always a useful basis for determining nursing actions because it leaves out many experiences that nurses and other health workers have to deal with nowadays. The crisis of a first day of school is not really an illness, yet, if not handled judiciously, it may lead to one (16). Having to learn how to get into one's girdle after one has had a stroke, or being thrown first up and then down by the moods of one's cyclothymic personality, does not necessarily mean one is ill, or even convalescing, yet one is badly in need of help in learning how to live within the confines of one's limitations. By sustaining the patient in his experience, the nurse can perhaps help to make bearable, to some degree, that which without her intervention might have been intolerable for him. We know that she cannot take his experience upon herself, but perhaps she can find measures to alleviate it or to help him bear it by lending him strength through her thereness. Perhaps, too, she can help him to make use of the experience in his own personal growth. In other words, she can aid him in coping with the elements of his current situation; her help and his coping will be accomplished at the rate, depth and effectiveness of which she and he are capable at the time.

"Experience" defined

At this point, perhaps it would be well for me to define the terms "experience" and "sustaining" and to illustrate these definitions by examples.

By "experience" I mean a certain process which occurs in a human being when he encounters an inner or outer event, another person, a living being, or a material object (17). Experience can be broken down into three phases: 1) One *perceives* an encounter in light of his physiological capacity, cultural conditioning and present knowledge; 2) one *interprets* the perceived encounter, again in light of his past experience and his present ability and knowledge; and 3) one *responds* to the encounter in accordance with his interpretation in ways that are opened to him by his capacity, his cultural heritage, and the framework of the given situation. The response may, in turn, be the beginning of a new experiential sequence.

A patient may have a deficiency or lack of skill in dealing with one or another of the phases of an "experience." He may have difficulty in perceiving because he lacks one of the essential senses, such as vision or hearing. He may perceive correctly, but may distort what he perceives because of his high level of anxiety, or because of faulty thinking patterns which he has not learned to correct. Also, the patient may perceive and interpret quite well but, due to a paralysis of his limbs or vocal cords, or overwhelming emotional conflict, he may not be able to respond adequately to the interpreted perception. In the case of unconscious, severely brain-damaged or extremely anxious patients, capacities for dealing with all three phases of the experience may be absent for a time.

"Sustaining" defined

This is an over-all term that covers all of the nurse's interventions that are designed to help the patient cope with or profit from his experience or to make adjustment for any one of the three components of experience that he lacks. First of all, it means acknowledging to oneself and to the patient that his experience, whatever it may be, is real to him. It may mean also providing that information which the patient needs, because he lacks in one or the other of his capacities to perceive; helping the patient learn to make corrections for his tendency to interpret his perception in a merely subjective way without taking objective facts into account (*see* Chapter 1); teaching the patient better or even new ways of communicating in case he cannot respond by ordinary means; and anticipating all needs of those patients who cannot perceive, interpret or respond. Sustaining the patient may mean such active intervention on the nurse's part as altering his position; giving him pain-relieving medication; calling the doctor; asking the patient to focus his attention on a concrete task in order to reduce his panic; helping him to tolerate his state by lending him some of her own strength, as it were; staying with him and thus reducing his fear; letting him be the way he can be, or wants to be, at any given time and thus conserving his energy by reducing his need to defend himself against external demands in addition to having to cope with his condition.

Sustaining the patient may also mean helping him to go beyond merely tolerating his experience in order to help him to direct his energy, if and when he can do so, into examining, understanding and overcoming the experience, and integrating it into his future life.

In Part III of this book we shall attempt to give a broader and more systematic presentation of what we mean by "sustaining the patient in his experience." Since the experience of another person cannot be assessed directly, we will give ways of approximating what the experience might be like for the patient. That is, we will examine factors that can be derived from the dynamics of the patient's condition, the meaning this condition may have for him, and his behavior—any one or all of which may give us leads as to his experience and the appropriate steps for sustaining him in it. In the meantime, let us look at a few examples to get an idea of some of the forms that sustaining a patient in his experience might take.

A nurse who is assisting a physician with a pelvic examination notes that the patient is very tense and that this makes it difficult for the physician to palpate her organs. He asks the patient to breathe deeply so that he can go on with the examination. The nurse does not simply reinforce the physician's request by restating that the patient should try to relax by means of deep breathing, but instead, she focuses on the patient's experience of undergoing an uncomfortable procedure. Therefore, she may give the patient an opportunity to hold on to her hand. Or, she may tell the patient that it will be less painful, and over sooner, if she will take several deep breaths now. The nurse may even breathe deeply a few times herself to help the patient get started.

A psychiatrist is touching upon some very upsetting material in working therapeutically with a patient diagnosed as alcoholic. As a result, the patient has become extremely anxious. He is frantic to get out of the hospital so that he can have a drink and feel better. Since the patient is in therapy, the nurse will not attempt to explore, on her own, the problem that disturbs him so, nor will she glibly tell him that if he drinks, his doctor cannot help him. Instead, she will stay (or offer to stay) with him while he is so anxious, and she may invite him to talk about his state if he wants to do so. (This is different from exploring the problem underlying his state.) She may offer him a cup of coffee, or a soft drink, and cookies in order to help relieve his oral cravings. Or, she may just sit silently, where he can see her, while he paces up and down the hall.

A public health nurse makes a call on an old lady who has recently had a hip pinning. On her arrival, the nurse is told that the doctor wants the lady out of bed but that she refuses to obey this order. The nurse introduces herself and tells the patient she has come to help her get up, and the old lady goes into a tirade against the doctor and clings to the bedrails as though her life depended on them. In light of the patient's terrific fear and her resistance to being moved, the nurse telephones the doctor and tells him that the patient will need a little time to prepare herself for getting out of bed. She stays a while with the patient and gives her care in bed so that the lady can get to know her and develop confidence in her skill. She also gradually explores, with the patient, what it is that frightens her so. Usually, a patient who clings to the bed, as this one does, has a deep fear of falling and of motion in general (a common phenomenon among older people). Therefore, the nurse will *very slowly* help the patient to get used to some motion and, at the same time, she will demonstrate that she is able to give the patient adequate, safe support. A few days later, it may be possible for her to suggest that the patient will soon be able to get out of bed and sit for a while in her easy chair. The chances are good that before very long the patient will not only be able to get up but, what is more, she probably will not be too averse to taking this major step.

Had there been serious need for the patient to get out of bed right away because of an impending lung congestion, for instance, the nurse might not have been able to proceed as slowly as she did. Although she would have acknowledged to the patient that she was aware of her fear of motion, and that she respected it, she would have had to exert considerable pressure on the patient to get her to comply with the doctor's order. Whether the nurse would have been successful in this case, we do not know. It might have helped had she been called in earlier, before the order had been given to get the patient out of bed. That would have given her the opportunity to anticipate the move and to rehearse it mentally, together with the patient, long before it became an impending actuality (18).

In each of these three examples, the nurse's primary concern was to sustain the patient in the particular experience he was undergoing. Neither facilitating the physician's work (as in the first case of the woman undergoing a pelvic examination), nor health teaching (as in the case of the alcoholic patient), nor following the doctor's orders (as in the third example) were primary considerations in the care the nurse gave. Yet, because she focused on the patient's subjective experience, the gynecologist's task was facilitated and the patient's discomfort cut short; the alcoholic patient was helped to endure his anxiety, and thus was brought a step closer to realizing that there are other means of coping with his problem than drinking; and, in the case of the old lady, the doctor's order was followed eventually (even though not at the exact time he might have wished), and without damaging the patient's self-esteem.

Would the outcomes have been the same if the nurse had concentrated primarily on carrying out the doctor's instructions, or on upholding hospital rules or health standards? Perhaps, but what would this have cost the patient in terms of energy and integrity?

Suppose we accept, for the time being, the idea that the focus of nursing is to be the sustaining of the patient (and his family) in his experience. What does this imply for the nurse's work within a given setting?

Nursing actions that sustain the patient

One implication may be that the nurse, even when very busy, will not treat the patient as an object of her care but rather she will consider him as a being with an "I," even when he is unconscious. It is her sensitivity to his experience (extending, of course, to those who are close to him) that will cause her to drape the patient even if he cannot perceive that he is being exposed, and that will keep her from discussing matters concerning him in his presence unless she plans to include him in the talk. Awareness of her primary concern will help her to gain the necessary strength to withstand the pressure of the setting that puts both her and the patient on an assembly line. Together with her peers, she can assist in helping to streamline many of the patient services, but she should insist that interpersonal contacts not be automated—that they be allotted all the time they need. Granted, she can teach in a group setting rather than instructing each patient by himself, if this seems indicated. But even so, each individual is entitled to the time it may take to prepare him for group learning, and for any questions he may wish to ask in private, afterwards.

The fact that the nurse's chief concern is with her client's subjective state does not imply, by any means, that she is not to be concerned with the objective world but quite the opposite. If the patient's experience is important to her, she will also attach importance to well-cared-for instruments and well-executed procedures. She cannot help but be concerned with the right diameter and sharpness of the needles she uses and with the site she, or someone she supervises, selects for the injection of a drug.

Of course, she will be concerned with the smooth running of the hospital and with conserving materials and the physician's equanimity and strength, but she will not give these concerns priority over her patient's needs. Should she have to decide between the institution and the physician on one hand and the patient on the other, she will know where she ought to stand. If, in order to make a patient comfortable, she has to use extra pads or gowns, she will not be too troubled about what this might do to the economics of the hospital. Regretfully, but unhesitatingly, she may have to waken an exhausted intern for the tenth time if the condition of the patient requires it.

Those nurses who have not already done so could benefit from browsing through Florence Nightingale's *Notes on Nursing* in which the author discusses a multiplicity of nursing activities. None of these activities are carried out for the sake of hygiene, cleanliness or nutrition per se; all are linked closely and purposefully to the experience of the patient.

Is all this talk about the patient's experience, and about the nurse supporting him in it, really necessary? Aren't they both self-evident and obvious? I wonder. Many practicing nurses identify as their chief concern the setting in which they operate, whether this be a hospital ward, industrial plant, or doctor's office. They are devoted to keeping things running smoothly and will let nothing interfere with that, least of all the patient. Other nurses are so interested in medical procedures that they may "hush" a patient so they can better observe the doctor's work. They may become so engrossed in learning how to flick the switch on an electric-shock machine, or how to insert a needle into a patient's vein, that they forget that attached to this switch may be a terrified patient who thinks he will be killed by electricity, or that at the end of the searching needle are nerve endings which are quite susceptible to pain. It may be deplorable for a physician to be so engrossed in the pathology of his patient that he forgets about the person suffering from it. This is a matter he may have to take up with his conscience, his profession, and his patient. If it is true, however, that the nurse's core concern is the sustaining of the patient in his experience, she cannot permit herself to be sidetracked by intellectual curiosity, loyalty to the institution or her need to master a new skill.

References

1. Morritt, Walter. "Psychology and the Trained Nurse," *Amer. J. Nursing* 9 (June, 1909), pp. 647-651.
2. Lesnick, Milton, and Anderson, Bernice. *Nursing Practice and the Law* (2nd ed.). Philadelphia: J. B. Lippincott Co., 1962.
3. Goodrich, Annie. *The Social and Ethical Significance of Nursing*. New York: The Macmillan Co., 1932, p. 51.
4. Pennock, Meta Rutter (ed.). *Makers of Nursing History*. New York: Lakeside Publications, 1928.
5. Nightingale, Florence. *Notes on Nursing*. London: Harrison, 1860. Facsimile reprinted by the University of Pennsylvania, 1965.
6. Harmer, Bertha. *Textbook of the Principles and Practice of Nursing* (5th ed.). New York: The Macmillan Co., 1955.
7. Holmes, Marguerite, and Werner, Jean A. *Psychiatric Nursing in a Therapeutic Community*. New York: The Macmillan Co., 1966.
8. Orlando, Ida Jean. *The Dynamic Nurse-Patient Relationship*. New York: G. P. Putnam's Sons, 1961.

9. Wiedenbach, Ernestine. *Clinical Nursing, a Helping Art.* New York: Springer Publishing Co., 1964.
10. Norris, Catherine, and Lohr, Mary. "Philosophy Underlying Integration of Psychiatric Nursing Concepts Throughout Basic Nursing Curriculums" in *Psychiatric Nursing Concepts and Basic Nursing Education.* Proceedings of the Conference at Boulder, Colo., June, 1959. New York: The National League for Nursing, 1960, pp. 7-44.
11. Peplau, Hildegard E. *Interpersonal Relations in Nursing.* New York: G. P. Putnam's Sons, 1952.
12. Travelbee, Joyce. *Interpersonal Aspects of Nursing.* Philadelphia: F. A. Davis Co., 1966.
13. Rogers, Martha E. *Educational Revolution in Nursing.* New York: The Macmillan Co., 1961.
14. American Nurses' Association. "First Position Paper on Education for Nursing." *Amer. J. Nursing 65* (Dec., 1965), pp. 106-111.
15. Nightingale, Florence. *op. cit.*, p. 75.
16. Caplan, Gerald (ed.). *Prevention of Mental Disorders in Children.* New York: Basic Books, 1961.
17. Ujhely, Gertrud B. "Basic Considerations for Nurse-Patient Interaction in the Prevention and Treatment of Emotional Disorders," *Nursing Clinics of N. America 1* (June, 1966), pp. 179-186.
18. Caplan, Gerald (ed.). *op. cit.*

Suggested Readings

Bacala, Jesus C. *The Professionalization of Nursing.* U. S. T. Press, operated by Novel Publishing Co., 1959.

Fairchild, L. McCarthy. "Discussion of Papers by Fernandez and Zagorin" in Proceedings of the Boulder, Colo. conference (see Reference 10 above).

Fuerst, Elinor, and Wolff, E. LuVerne. *Fundamentals of Nursing.* Philadelphia: J. B. Lippincott Co., 1956, Foreword and Chapters 1-3.

Lounsbery, Harriet Camp. "The Nurse as a Teacher," *Amer. J. Nursing 12* (April, 1912), pp. 550-553.

Peplau, Hildegard E. "Specialization in Professional Nursing," *Nursing Science 3* (Aug., 1965), pp. 268-287.

Reiter, Frances. "The Nurse-Clinician," *Amer. J. Nursing 66* (Feb., 1966), pp. 274-280.

Simms, Laura. "The Clinical Nurse Specialist: An Experiment," *Nursing Outlook 13* (Aug., 1965), pp. 26-28.

Smith, Dorothy W., and Gips, Claudia. *The Care of the Adult Patient* (2nd ed.). Philadelphia: J. B. Lippincott Co., 1966.

Stonsby, Ella V. "This I Believe . . . About the Why of Collegiate Education in Nursing," *Nursing Outlook 15* (May, 1967), pp. 49-51.

Whiting, Leila, and Whiting, Joseph F. "Finding the Core of Hospital Nursing," *Amer. J. Nursing 62* (Aug., 1962), pp. 80-83.

Chapter 7

The Relationship Itself

For the remainder of our discussion of the nurse-patient relationship, we shall assume that the nurse is primarily concerned with sustaining her clients in their subjective experiences. The *how* of this sustaining action depends, apart from the client's individual state and the nurse's competency in the field, on a variety of factors, such as the phase of development of the relationship, its duration and the frequency with which it occurs, and, last but not least, the setting in which nurse and patient find themselves. Although these factors are closely interrelated, for the sake of clarity they will be discussed separately. Let us turn first to the phases of the nurse-patient relationship.

Customarily, one can distinguish three developmental phases of a relationship: the orientation phase; the working phase; and the termination phase. Each phase provides certain guidelines for the nurse's actions.

The Orientation Phase

During the *orientation* phase it is of paramount importance that the nurse pay careful attention to what the patient says because it is then that he outlines the area concerning which he is asking for help. Also, the orientation phase serves, to a great extent, as the model for the later phases.

During the orientation phase the nurse as the professional

person sets the outer limits of the relationship, while what happens within these limits is largely determined by the patient (client). In other words, the nurse introduces herself to the patient, lets him know when, for how long and how often she will be with him, and to what purpose. Within this given framework the patient is free to proceed at his own pace and in the direction of his choice.

Here are three examples of how the nurse-patient relationship may develop during the orientation phase. Suppose a patient comes to a general hospital. He is scheduled to have a hernia operation the next day. The nurse introduces herself and also the aide who is to take him to his room. Soon thereafter the nurse goes to his room to see whether there is anything he needs at the moment, and offers to orient him as to what he may expect to happen before and after the operation. She tells him how much time she has available for him at the moment and assures him that she can come again if more time should be needed for their talk. The patient may, or may not, take her up on her offer to orient him. If he does, she encourages him to stop her at any point to ask questions or make comments. Given this opportunity, the patient is likely to ask questions about those areas which are of most concern to him. Will he get a sleeping tablet? Will he come back to the same room after the operation? Will his wife be allowed to see him? The nurse answers his questions to the best of her ability and proceeds with her orientation only after she has received a cue from the patient that he is ready to go on. Perhaps she is not able to cover all pertinent material in the time available to her. In that case, she will let him know that she has to leave, but that she will be back in an hour, or whatever time period, so that they may continue their talk. Before she goes off duty, she lets the patient know when he can expect her to return and who will be taking care of him in her absence.

Another example involves a visiting nurse who goes to see a family that has never been seen by anyone from her agency. Before she can proceed with the business for which she was called in, she must, according to agency policy, assess the family's financial status. She needs to make this point very clear in her orientation, and ask her questions openly, rather than sneaking them in without the family's awareness that their finances are being assessed. Only if she is frank and forthright with them can she expect them to gradually lose the fear that she might make use of their statements for purposes for which they had not intended them to be used.

A third example involves a psychiatric nurse who has been assigned to work closely with a particular patient. The nurse and patient have known each other superficially for several weeks, ever since the patient came to the ward, but until now they have not had a counseling relationship. This nurse does not need to introduce herself to the patient. She does, however, have to explain to him the framework and nature of their future interviews. She lets the patient know, therefore, that she will be with him every day from 1:00 to 2:00 P.M. for the next four weeks except on her days off, that they will meet in his room, and that this time is set aside for him to talk about his present concerns as he sees them. Note the focus of the interviews could also have been for him to talk about himself, about his plans concerning his discharge, or what not. What is important is that the patient be given a focus and a framework within which he can feel free to proceed as he wishes. He is also entitled to know with whom the nurse will share the information he gives her and whether he may attend these interviews on a voluntary basis or whether he is required to participate.

Setting the focus for the interaction

From the examples given earlier, it can be seen that the width of focus for the discussion depends on the over-all purpose of the nurse-patient meeting. If it takes place for the sake of giving a specific treatment, teaching a specific skill or gaining specific information, the nurse sets a relatively narrow focus. In counseling interviews the focus is usually kept wider; for instance, the patient is encouraged to talk about himself, his present concerns or his current experience.

Even though the nurse sets the over-all focus for their interaction, she may find that the patient, whom she is perhaps just meeting for the first time, is unable to keep to this focus. His anxiety level may be so high, for instance, that he is unable to absorb the teaching offered by the nurse. In this case, the nurse may have to readjust the focus of the interview to suit the patient's present state. Of course, she has to explain this readjustment in clear terms and must give him the reasons for it as well. For example, she may have to say to him in so many words that, even though she had told him originally that she would teach him how to irrigate his bladder, it may be better for him if they first both considered his present state of unrest because until this condition is resolved, he is not likely to retain all the details of the procedure.

Many nurses are reluctant to clearly state a change in the focus of their interaction with a patient even though such readjustment is indicated at the time. They seem to be afraid that, if they change their minds, the patient will think them unreliable, ignorant or foolish. Yet, these same nurses are often unnecessarily inconsistent with their patients and are frequently not even aware of it. For example, such a nurse may ask a patient to tell her about himself. The patient, trying to think of something worth telling her, is silent for a while. The nurse becomes uneasy during this silence. In order to "get him to talk," she asks him questions about what he had for lunch today or whether his family has visited him lately. Now the patient becomes bewildered. Why did she change the subject? Is she annoyed because he took so long to answer her first question? He hurries to answer the second one and waits, wondering what she might want to know next. The nurse asks another question. The patient answers. Silence. Another question from the nurse–and so on. What is it that has happened to the interview, and that has probably also set the pattern for all subsequent interviews? The nurse has received answers to her questions, but the patient was not given an opportunity to tell her about himself in the way she originally indicated, the way he wanted to tell her or at his own rate of speed.

Here is another example of inconsistency on the part of the nurse who is setting the stage for an interaction. A visiting nurse is seeing a diabetic patient for the purpose of teaching him how to administer insulin to himself. Before she starts with the actual instruction, she encourages the patient to ask any questions he might have about giving himself these injections. The patient replies, "No, you ask me questions and I will answer." The nurse complies with his request, but will her questions necessarily tap the area about which he wants, or needs, to get more information?

What has happened here is that the nurse has probably forgotten that whenever limits are established by one of the partners in a relationship, the other is liable to test these limits to see whether they are really firm before he will entrust himself to them. Often the nurse is intimidated by these testing maneuvers and, before she realizes what is happening, the limits are broken down. What trust can the patient have in a relationship whose boundaries crumble at his first, feeble assault? "Well," the nurse will say, "I did not want to be caught in a power struggle with him." This is a laudable intent indeed, for there is practically nothing more futile or wasteful of energy than a power struggle between human beings. The nurse does not really need to enter into such a struggle, however. Instead, she can take the patient up on his comment and discuss it with him. She can try to find out whether she failed to make herself clear in the first place, which is quite possible. She can also try to find out why the patient objects to talking about himself. Perhaps he is not used to it. Well, he can learn—there is time. He may not want to talk to her; this fact needs to be respected, if he really means it. The nurse will usually know whether he does mean it or not from the other behavioral clues that he gives her simultaneously with his spoken refusal and, possibly, from her prior experience with patients who were in some way similar to him.

Setting the limits of the relationship

Many patients cannot grasp the framework the nurse sets for their interaction the first time she states it. They may not be used to the patient role, or they may not have had previous experience with nurses setting such a framework. Also, their anxiety level may be high so that any statement, unless it is particularly meaningful to them within the context of their current preoccupation, is rarely fully heard, much less fully integrated, the first time around. Even people who choose, on their own, to undergo psychotherapy may, after months or years of treatment, ask their therapist what they are really supposed to do in this relationship, even though they have been told the limits of the relationship not merely once, but many times. In fact, once the patient assumes responsibility to uphold these limits by himself, he is no longer in the orientation phase but has already entered into the working phase of the relationship. But more about that later. What is important here is that the nurse must either repeat her statements about the framework of the relationship several times (and in different words) or at least keep her finger on the pulse of the situation in order to know whether or not the patient understands the framework as she described it.

Many nurses object to what appears to be a rigid structuring of the relationship because they think it stifles spontaneity on the nurse's (and the patient's) part. Individuals are different from each other, they say, and, therefore, each patient should be treated differently. Besides, the patient should use the nurse's time as he sees fit and not be hampered by boundaries she may set for him.

Of course individuals are different. It takes time to get to know them, however, and it is best that each unfold himself to the other person at his own pace. Would it be better if the nurse prodded the patient with questions based on her own individual interests in order to get him to tell her everything she wants to know about him? This happens quite often, by the way. Not knowing what to say to the stranger in front of her, the nurse will try to keep the conversation going by asking him where he lives, whether he is married, has any children, what his likes and dislikes are, and so on. She does not do this to get information for an intake form, mind you, but just to "get to know the patient." Does she really get to know him this way? The patient answers her questions as laconically as he can, and wishes that she would stop questioning him so that he can concentrate long enough to formulate in his mind what it is that bothers him and then put it into words.

The nurse's manner should be as matter-of-fact as possible during this orientation period, for she does not know the patient and his idiosyncrasies. Even a smile on her part could easily be interpreted by him as a sign of ridicule or pity, either one of which he may abhor. But she can express some individuality in the tone of voice she uses, the choice of words she makes, the kind of attention she devotes to him.

Suppose the nurse does not set limits for her relationship with the patient but lets him use her time the way he sees fit—"according to his needs." Suppose he takes her up on this and asks her for a date? Or, suppose he asks the only nurse on the ward to stay in his room during the next hour or so because he is lonely and wants someone to talk to? The nurse will then have to clarify the nature and the limitations of their relationship, what is acceptable and possible within these, and what is not, but, in the meantime, has she not allowed much of her patient's energy to be wasted in this trial and error exploration? Is it possible that such hit-or-miss exploration of the limits of the relationship may also be the cause of unpleasant damage to the patient's self-esteem? Does she not show more respect for the patient as a person if she gives him the "rules of the game" of this new relationship that he has entered? Must he be burdened with the task of having to find out about it for himself in addition to already being burdened with his new and often painful patient role?

The point is that there must be boundaries for every interaction between human beings, whether or not we are consciously aware of them. They are established by the roles of the people who are relating to each other and by the norms set up in each society for the performance of these roles (*see* Chapter 5). Of course, there is room for individual variation within each role because, as we said earlier, no two individuals are alike.

In her private life, the nurse may not always be conscious of the norms for the various relationships she is engaged in, but she observes them just the same. For example, she would not think of monopolizing the other girl's boy friend while on a double date, or applying the rules of baseball to a tennis game. Just so, in her professional relationships it behooves her to be consciously mindful of her role and of those of the people with whom she interacts. It also behooves her to facilitate awareness of these roles in her clients, because if she does not help them explicitly, those to whom the roles are new may have to get the information through other channels, either by trial and error, as we have described above, or through other people who have already arrived at some conclusions, not all of which are necessarily correct. Thus, one patient may inform his new neighbor she is "too busy." And if he must call her, he had better apologize for taking up her time.

The patient's contribution to the orientation phase

We said that in the orientation phase the patient, if given half a chance, will outline for the nurse the area he would like to discuss with her. He may do this clearly and intentionally. Or, he may not be aware of the fact that he has a problem or that he has just let the nurse look in on it. The latter happens particularly with patients who are distraught by acute or long-standing pain, anxiety or conflict. Such patients are likely to make several apparently unrelated statements that do not appear to hang together as far as their content is concerned. Yet, they do hang together—not logically perhaps—but through association or through their affects. If the nurse lets herself hear what the patient says and how he says it, she will soon get an idea of the key concepts or key ideas which underlie his statements and which bind them together into dim, but discernible shape. She will then become aware of three kinds of underlying key ideas, or *themes*, as we call them from now on: the *content* theme (or themes); the *mood* theme; and the theme of *interaction*.

Themes of the interaction

When a patient tells the nurse that he is quite worried about the fact that he has had a relapse, he may be implying that he fears his insurance will run out before he is discharged from the hospital or that his employer will no longer hold his job for him. The content theme underlying this communication may be called, until it gets further delineation, financial insecurity.

While the nurse listens to the theme underlying the *what* of the patient's communication, she also listens to *how* he gets it across to her. Does he seem frightened? In this case, the mood theme may be fear or even anxiety, i.e., fear of the unknown. Does he seem weepy, sorry for himself? In that case, the theme may be self-pity, grief, or perhaps depression. Does he seem defiant? Perhaps then the mood theme is anger or frustration.

As the patient continues talking, the nurse will either be confirmed in her hunch as to the underlying themes, or she may realize that she has to revise her original assumption. The chances are that if she really listens to what the patient says and how he comes across to her, she will not go very far wrong in picking up his themes. She must guard against seeking to find the *cause* of the patient's problem prematurely, however, for the cause will become apparent only after all the facts are in. By listening for the cause of the problem, she may miss hearing what the patient is trying to communicate to her.

Further, it is important that the nurse note in what way the patient behaves in relation to her. Does he even notice that she is there, that she is a real person? Does he ignore her comments? Does he ask her to tell him what to do, as if she had all the answers? His behavior toward her and—just as important—her response to it, constitute the interaction theme. A variety of interaction themes occur. It is important that the nurse not allow herself to be provoked into behavior complementary to that of the patient, unless this is desirable for the subsequent development of the relationship. For example, a patient in a psychiatric unit interacts with the nurse in a submissive way: He asks the nurse whether he may go to the fountain for a drink of water. The nurse must be careful that she does not, unthinkingly, fall into the complementary dominant behavior by stating, "Yes, of course, you may." Originally, she gave the patient freedom within the limits she set up and she must not violate this freedom now, even though, for the moment, a role complementarity on her part may be more comfortable for him. Instead, she should remind him that she will be there for the time stated and let him know that it is entirely up to him whether he wants to have his drink of water now or afterwards.

Or, the patient may start to reminisce about old times. This may easily evoke memories in the nurse as well. She must refrain, however, from reminiscing too, in a "parallel-play" attitude, not really focused on the patient. Instead, she must be alert to the connections between his reminiscences and his present plight.

It would appear to be relatively simple to allow the patient to develop his themes during the orientation phase, yet it is quite common for nurses to interfere, unwittingly, with this development rather than helping it along. This interference usually takes place in one or more of the following ways: The nurse latches on to the first statement the patient makes and pursues it in detail; in her eagerness to hear the full story, the nurse hurries his account along; or, for fear of making the wrong comment, the nurse says nothing at all, and the patient, not getting any reinforcement, slows down in his communication and gradually extinguishes its flow (1). Let us discuss briefly each of these quite common errors.

The patient may open the conversation by saying, "My brother and I went to Coney Island." Now, the nurse has no idea what he is driving at. He has given her an opening but, as yet, she cannot possibly guess his themes. All she really needs to do to encourage him in some way to go on is to let him know she has heard him and that she will continue to listen. She can do this in one of many ways—by nodding, by saying "hm, hm," by saying "Yes, go on," by saying nothing at all but looking attentive. What nurses frequently do, however, is to grasp this first, ambiguous statement and concentrate on it by asking such questions as: "How old is your brother?" "Where is Coney Island?" "Did you drive there?" "When was that?" Now, these questions may well be in order when the proper time for asking them comes, but that time has not yet come. Perhaps the patient is only using this sentence as an introduction to telling her about what happened to him on that particular day, i.e., he almost drowned. If his trend of thought is deflected by her premature, too narrow questioning, he will need an extraordinary amount of courage to stop her and tell her that he does not want to talk about his brother, or the road to Coney Island, but merely about his accident.

As to the second error, suppose a patient in a home for the aged and infirm tells the nurse that she was in an orphanage from the time she was three years old until she was six. Instead of letting the patient know in some way that she has heard her, the nurse asks, "And then what happened?" The patient answers by telling the nurse that afterwards her father remarried and she was taken back home. But the point she had been trying to make had to do with the period during which she was in the orphanage —a period which had many similarities with her present situation.

Some nurses seem to have been taught that during the orientation phase the nurse must not make any comments, especially not ask questions. The following incident is a case in point. A rather agitated woman, diagnosed as having a schizophrenic reaction, chronic undifferentiated type, told the nurse a long, complicated story involving many different people who were not identified and places that were not called by name. Early in this tangled account, the nurse lost her bearings, but she did not dare to interrupt the patient for clarification. Instead, she kept quiet, trying hard not to let her bewilderment show. In fact, she did not even allow herself to nod or make listening noises, since she was not quite sure where these might fit in. The patient completed her story and then lapsed into silence. Nurse and patient looked at each other for several minutes. Finally, the patient got up, said that she had told the nurse all there was to tell and walked away. She never talked with that particular nurse again.

The outcome of this incident points out why the nurse is not only permitted, but actually obliged, to ask the patient to clarify his statements if she cannot follow them. In fact, if she asks him to whom he is referring when he says "we" or "they" or "he," the nurse shows him a great deal more respect than if she humors him, as one might a small child, and pretends she understands.

It is important then, that during the orientation phase the nurse be not merely a passive listener, but that she listen in such a way as to help the patient to delineate the territory of his concern.

The Working Phase

How long does the orientation phase take and at what point does the working phase begin? Usually, the transition from one phase to the next is gradual. It rarely happens all at once. When there is prolonged and frequent contact between nurse and patient, and when the patient is reasonably alert and well motivated, the orientation phase will take up the time of two or three meetings. If the patient is very anxious, however, or very ill, or if he has suffered brain damage, the relationship may never progress beyond the initial stage. Or, if nurse and patient have only one opportunity to meet, in the emergency or operating room, for instance, time may not permit more than "Hello" and "Good-bye" (*see* Chapter 8). Sometimes, especially if the patient has been exposed to therapeutic relationships before, he may proceed into the working phase as soon as the limits of the relationship have been spelled out to him.

Characteristics of the working phase

What characterizes the working phase of the nurse-patient relationship? Generally speaking, it is during this phase that the patient fills in the territory he has outlined for the nurse during the orientation period and begins to come to grips with his experience. The nurse facilitates this filling-in process by directing the patient's attention to areas that are still hazy. She also helps him with gathering the tools he needs for coping with the experience that confronts him.

How does the nurse recognize that the patient has reached the working phase? First, she observes that he has largely accepted most of the boundaries she gave him concerning their relationship and that he no longer needs to test them out. Therefore, he is devoting his energy increasingly to what goes on *within* these boundaries, i.e., to mapping out his problem area in detail. Secondly, and more concretely, the nurse observes that the patient is expecting her arrival, is waiting and ready for their talk. He has begun to keep track of their time together and frequently apprizes the nurse of the topic he wishes to take up with her. Usually this topic will be one of those he has mentioned, in passing, during the orientation phase. Further, he is increasingly able to give the nurse a description of the subject under discussion, that is, he highlights it from various angles of approach with respect to time sequence and location, and in relation to what he has discussed before. In addition, he has learned to clarify his statements without prior prompting by the nurse, he substitutes proper names for pronouns in cases of ambiguity, and he may pause occasionally to ask the nurse whether he has made himself clear.

In the beginning of the working phase, however, the patient still needs considerable help from the nurse in learning how to gain fuller awareness of what it is that really troubles him about the episodes he had outlined to her during the period of orientation. He needs the nurse's judicious questions to help him to enlarge upon his descriptions so that gradually a complete picture can emerge. If this help is not forthcoming, he may tend to go over the same story the same way as he did before, without getting much relief from it, or any deeper understanding. It is important, therefore, that the nurse not merely listen to him, but that she actively steer his inquiry so that he may obtain as complete a picture as possible of the topic upon which he has embarked.

"But which topic?" the nurse may well ask, for the patient may have touched upon a number of topics during the orientation phase. It will be helpful if the nurse suggests discussing first those topics that make up the patient's *content* theme (or themes). That is, she may refer him to an incident he had discussed during their previous conversation and ask him to tell her exactly—blow by blow—what happened. Or, she may ask, "What did you do when you were told . . .?" "When was this?" (2).

The mood theme

When the patient has fully described the various events, actions and thoughts that surround the theme, he will be able to identify and name the theme in question, either by himself, or aided by the nurse. Only then should his attention be drawn to the *mood* theme associated with his account. When it comes to the mood theme, however, the nurse cannot always expect the patient to describe immediately the relevant points surrounding it. Often she must first help him to *observe* the mood or feeling tone in question, i.e., to become aware of its existence, because it is not possible to describe something that one does not know exists, or something one is afraid to face and therefore must deny. It is even less possible for one to get at the reason for one's unnoticed feelings, or to deal with them constructively.

Why should the nurse steer her inquiry first to the content theme and only then in the direction of the patient's feeling? And when does she deal with the theme of interaction?

In our culture, people tend to find it easier to discuss events, actions and thoughts than to reveal their deeper feelings. Also, the mood theme is, in most instances, contingent upon the events which happened in the patient's life and his experience of them (i.e., his perception, interpretation, and response). Hence, neither nurse nor patient may get very far in a discussion of his feelings if they are unable to relate them to the circumstances of his life. Unfortunately, nurses often deal prematurely with their patients' feeling state and, as a result, they must resort to all kinds of speculation as to what may be the cause of the feelings. Needless to say, such speculation does little to help resolve the patient's plight.

The interaction theme

What, then, about the interaction theme? We have stressed that the nurse should keep close watch over what goes on between herself and her patient. It is true that she must be alert to patterns in their interaction, so that she does not unwittingly fall into a complementary role which may be detrimental to the patient's growth. She does not need to draw his attention to this theme, however, unless it has specific meaning for the subject matter at hand, or unless a barrier has developed between them that may make further joint enquiry difficult.

One may ask, "Why should the patient's attention not be drawn much more frequently to how he behaves in the nurse-patient situation? After all, the chances are that his interaction with the nurse is merely an example of his habitual behavior." This point is well taken, and the answer is that the nurse's task consists in helping the patient with a particular experience and is not usually concerned with helping him to revise his personality. But suppose the nurse allows the relationship itself to become the center of her discussion with her client. What will happen to the usually manageable quantity of transference phenomena between them, i.e., the attribution of qualities belonging to significant figures from the past to the other person in the current situation? The chances are that these transference phenomena will take on enormous proportions and, unless the nurse is also a trained psychotherapist, she is not equipped to deal with them. Then what happens? Most likely, the nurse or the patient, or both, will become so uncomfortable in the situation that they will have to pull away from it to obtain relief. It is very important, therefore, that in a nurse-patient relationship the transference be kept within reasonable bounds. To this end, the judicious nurse will deal with the interaction theme only if it is indicated within the larger context of their work together. If the patient chooses to delve into similarities between her and, say, his mother, she will help him to see the differences between them as well.

Progress of the interaction

As the working phase progresses and after the patient has given the nurse a rather full description of the experience with which he is concerned, the nurse will assist him to abstract the themes most significant for his situation and to look at the component parts of each theme. She shows him, further, how one can manipulate these parts to bring about the solution most appropriate to one's own life. Finally, the nurse, through patience and encouragement, sustains him as he tries out his new insights in the current situation and, from time to time, she reviews with him his application of these insights to new but similar life events.

Of course, there is no guarantee that nurse and patient will be able to go through this entire process during the working phase of their relationship. It may take all the time they have together to help the patient learn how to observe or to describe. Also, the patient's intellectual capacity may be so limited that he is unable to make abstractions from concrete situations. Or, his tolerance for anxiety may be so low, or his habit pattern so persistent that, although he has learned a great deal from their talks, he is still unable to utilize what they may have revealed.

This does not mean, however, that the nurse should be disappointed, or that she should take shortcuts in order to reach a final goal. It takes time to erect a building, and sometimes the building process may have to be halted for a while. As long as there is a solid foundation, however, the process can be resumed at a later and, hopefully, more auspicious, date. But if shortcuts were taken in laying the foundation, it may well be that much of what has been erected must be torn down and this would really represent unnecessary waste of time and energy.

The following examples show what a working relationship might look like in actual nursing practice:

A nurse is having biweekly counseling interviews with an adolescent girl on a ward for chronically ill mental patients. The patient had worked with various psychotherapists before her hospitalization and therefore it takes very little time for her to enter into the working phase.

Two main content themes emerge during the period of orientation: 1) unpredictable fits of anger, of which the patient is very much afraid, and which, in addition, lead to unpleasant punishment and sanctions from the ward personnel; and 2) in spite of the patient's great need to have friends, she seems to be unable to maintain friendships once she has established them.

The patient's mood fluctuates from despondency to fury, as, upon the nurse's prompting, she relates the details of the various incidents she has experienced.

At first, the patient pleads with the nurse to give her some formula by which she can stop these outbursts and also bind newly acquired friends to herself. The nurse points out to her that such a formula, even if there were such a thing, could only emerge after she and the patient have examined closely what actually occurs. After that, the patient collaborates diligently with her by giving a full description of each incident.

Before long, it becomes evident to the nurse that the patient's main theme binding content and mood together is *frustration*. That is, she tends to set her goals too high by making inordinate demands on the people whose friendship she desires. This is followed by withdrawal on their part. When the patient has no way of reaching the object of her efforts, the slightest, often unrelated provocation will send her into wild fits of rage or to moping despairingly in a corner.

It would be premature, however, to explain the theme of frustration to the patient before the girl has clearly seen it manifest itself. Therefore, the nurse asks the patient to pay particular attention not only to the incidents themselves and to the response of others, but also to her own part in them. After a few days, the patient tells her how, during the preceding night, while unable to sleep, she kept her roommate, whom she likes very much and considers her new friend, awake with long conversations. In the morning, the roommate avoided her and would have nothing to do with her. The nurse asks the patient if she would be willing to give up her own sleep just because a friend finds it easier to cope with sleeplessness by talking. The patient considers the question carefully and finally admits that she would not. "And yet you expect your friend to make this sacrifice for you?" the nurse asks.

In the course of the discussion it has also become apparent that the patient's mother is a rather ungiving, aloof person and that the girl feels that everything would be all right if only her mother would change. Although she listens to the patient, the nurse does not ask her to delve into this topic nor to enlarge on her wishful thoughts about it. One day, however, shortly before the nurse is to leave on a two weeks' vacation, the patient suddenly turns on her and, crying bitterly, blurts out, "You are just like my mother! You never had my interest at heart! Only your own pleasure! Just like my mother! But never mind, I really don't care whether you live or die. And I will certainly not talk to you again when you're back!"

The nurse waits calmly until this outburst of rage and self-pity blows over. Then, very quietly, she asks the patient to think about the following during her absence: What might be more useful for her in the long run—spending her energy in wishing she could get what the nurse does not have to give her, or taking full advantage of what the nurse does have to give, even though it may be less than she might like?

Upon her return she finds the patient, somewhat shamefacedly, waiting for her. When the patient asks her about her vacation she replies with a brief, general statement and turns to the question she had asked her to think about during their last talk. The patient does not answer her directly but tells her she has begun to see the connection between her temper outbursts and her expectations of other people. She can see now that she has wanted others to be different, to give her more than they had to offer and that she concentrated so much on what she could not get that what she did receive seemed hardly worth her while. She sees that perhaps it does make more sense in the long run to try to let others be the way they are, and to take—and expect—from them only what they have to offer, instead of getting all worked up about the way they could be and would be if only *they* would try.

Of course, it takes time to put ideational insights into practice, and the nurse, in turn, should not expect too much of her client. By-and-by, however, the patient is able to apply her new learning, first in the ward situation, then during her trial visits home. She learns to leave her friends alone when they don't want to be bothered, and to occupy herself, for short periods of time at least, with solitary tasks. She now also asks her mother, beforehand, whether she would mind if another patient came home with her, rather than expecting her mother to be a gracious hostess to unannounced, and sometimes rather bizarre, weekend visitors.

As might be expected, her mood swings have become less violent and do not occur as often; thus there is less need for curtailing her privileges. As might also be expected, she is able to keep friends for much longer periods than she could before. Even her relationship with her mother has become somewhat more relaxed and cordial, since her mother feels less pressure to give more than she has to offer.

The patient is not cured, of course, nor is she ready for living in the outside world. But she has been helped by the nurse to cope with one aspect of her experience and, as a result, is less frightened of herself and one step closer to recovery.

Here is another example of a working relationship between nurse and patient. Miss D. is suffering from a very painful metastatic cancer. In order to control the pain, she has been given large amounts of narcotic medication. Lately, however, it is more and more apparent that she has become addicted to the drugs. This might have been acceptable, had she been in the very last stages of her illness, but it so happens that, in spite of the metastatic nature of her disease, it has been possible to slow down its progress through some of the newer therapies. There is no telling at this time whether her life span has been increased by several months, or even longer. It is important, therefore, that attention be given to the problem of her addiction, in spite of the severe pain connected with her condition.

The physician explains the situation to the patient and her family. He points out to them that they will have to choose between a long period of lethargy, associated with addiction, and the hope that she might again take an interest in various aspects of her life, even though these activities would, at times, be accompanied by very severe pain. Before her illness, the patient—a very gifted woman—could find joy in a variety of topics and activities. Therefore, she and her family decide on the more painful course of action, so that she may be allowed to consciously participate in the lifetime still ahead of her. It is decided, therefore, to gradually withdraw the patient from the narcotics and to help her learn to tolerate her pain, aided merely by non-addictive analgesic drugs. Of course, it is one thing to arrive at such a decision and quite another to see it through, especially if it involves the patient's having to get rid of an addiction and, at the same time, having to tolerate severe pain.

The patient and her family will need all the support they can get. It is decided, therefore, to employ skilled and well-prepared private duty nurses who can sustain her during this crucial period and who also can work closely with one another in order to provide continuity of care. For the sake of clarifying the working phase of the nurse-patient relationship, the focus in the following discussion will not be on the contributions of each individual nurse, but rather we shall speak about their contributions as if they were all made by the same person.

After nurse and patient have worked out a general plan of action, the nurse asks the patient to concentrate on getting to know her pain. When does it occur? What are the circumstances which provoke it? It takes many days for the patient to come to grips with this request, since she is often overwhelmed not only by her suffering, but also by her need for the medication which will not only blot out the pain but the depressing fact of her illness as well. During such times of intense need, the patient becomes quite demanding and unreasonable. She sees the nurse as a heartless and cruel creature who wants to see her suffer. She refuses the non-narcotic medication the nurse offers and, in addition, calls her a variety of unflattering names. At such times, the nurse does not argue with the patient, respond in kind, or act offended. She simply stays with the patient until the attack exhausts itself. Afterwards, when the patient has had some rest, the nurse asks her to talk about what happened.

Gradually, it becomes clear that the patient is responding not only to the pain itself, but also to her fear of its occurring, should she make a wrong movement. It is her fear that the pain will get worse that makes her ask for the pain-relieving medication. Sometimes, thoughts about the illness itself, the certainty of its unfortunate outcome, and the unreasonableness that it should have befallen her—of all people—will translate themselves into pain and an urgent need for medication.

Under the nurse's guidance and support, the patient gradually learns to get to know her pain. She learns to differentiate it from fear and from despair; she learns to know when it will occur, the course it will take from its onset until its peak and eventual subsidence; she learns which movements will provoke it and which movements she can afford to make without having to suffer later. In this process of objectifying her pain, the patient has jokingly given it a name. She calls it Max and holds dialogues with it, asking it what it wants, telling it to stop hurting, or demanding that it let her be for just a little while.

The nurse respects the patient's suggestions as to when and how she should move her and when to leave her alone. She listens as the patient describes the pain, but does not, herself, focus on it when there is no occasion to do so. She leaves newspapers or books within the patient's reach, or she may read aloud a passage that she believes might interest the patient. She points out changes in the weather or in the foliage of the trees outside her window. She obtains permission to have a songbird brought to the patient's room.

Slowly the patient becomes able to occupy the time between painful periods more fully. She reads a little, sees an occasional visitor. She listens to music or watches the cloud patterns in the sky. The doctors are pleased with her progress. Everyone is proud of her, for not only has she been able to relinquish the narcotics altogether, but she now requires very few other non-narcotic, pain-relieving drugs. She is very ill, indeed, and suffering deeply from her illness. Yet, through her own strength, and the judicious support given by the three nurses who sustained her in her struggles day and night, she has learned to cope with her experience and to come to terms with it.

The Termination Phase

Whenever possible, the termination phase of the relationship ought not to be suddenly sprung on the patient during the last time the nurse meets with the patient. Instead, it should be built into the relationship from the very first day. That is, if the patient's condition indicates that the termination date for the interaction is at all foreseeable, this fact should be kept in mind and openly discussed at frequent intervals. This way, the patient has an opportunity to gauge how much he wants to share with the nurse in the time allotted. Also, the nurse is helped to decide whether she should encourage him to open up a new topic or whether, because of the lack of time available to them, it had better be looked at with someone else at a later date.

Usually, the last meeting of the nurse and patient is considered to be the "termination" proper. At this time, they summarize each of the areas discussed during their previous encounters, and evaluate the progress which has been made. The patient is given an opportunity to voice openly what he liked and disliked about their work together and to thank the nurse for the help she has given him. The nurse, in turn, lets the patient know that she, too, has received something from the relationship; through knowing the patient she too has learned and gained deeper insight, and will be a better nurse for it.

Sometimes, during the last session, a patient behaves as if the intervening meetings had never taken place. He may be just as distant or distrustful as he was at their first meeting. Or, he may bring up symptoms and fears which the nurse thought were long since taken care of and worked out. She need not be alarmed or discouraged by this phenomenon. Separation is not an easy event for anyone to accept, especially if one has come to know, like and respect the other person, or if one has had to go through many, often premature terminations of relationships for which one was not emotionally ready, or for which one was ill prepared. Even though the patient's behavior may seem like a plea to her not to let go of him (or even though the nurse may, herself, find it hard to accept the termination), it is important that the nurse be able to make a clean break. If she tries to keep up the relationship merely to lessen the patient's anxiety, she will find it burdensome, since it has lost its initial and real purpose. Later, she will have to get rid of it—in self-defense—or, if she keeps it up indefinitely, she will resent the patient for it more and more.

Some nurses find the termination phase especially difficult because they imagine the patient will never adjust to it. This is an unrealistic fear based on an overly strong need for being needed. He will get over the separation in due time, especially if he has been adequately prepared for it. After all, she is not the first person he has met nor will she be the last. Life provides new experiences continuously, and if the nurse has been at all instrumental in helping the patient to learn to make use of what life has to offer, she need not be unduly concerned.

It will be helpful for both patient and nurse, though, if, from the beginning of their relationship, the nurse gives the patient the opportunity to voice his thoughts and feelings concerning termination. Thus, over time, they can discuss together its meaning for the patient, instead of his having to deal with it alone, after it has occurred.

Some nurses are ashamed to admit that they, too, feel the pangs of separation. Why should they not feel them? Have they not invested a great deal of themselves in their work with the patient? Have they not come to know him rather well? Other nurses, especially those who have traveled a great deal and have worked here and there, never for very long periods, may not be strongly affected by terminating their relationships with patients. This does not mean that they are heartless or that they do not care; it simply means that they have had to learn to take separations in stride as part of their lives.

Perhaps now we can see more clearly how the nurse-patient relationship varies in accordance with each of its phases. After having been relatively matter-of-fact and not too personal in the orientation phase, the nurse becomes more and more the patient's guide and working partner until, toward the end of the relationship, she is very much a human being who has been privileged to provide, for a time, professional assistance to another person in need of her skill.

References

1. Verplanck, W. "The Control of the Content of Conversation: Reinforcement of Statements of Opinion," *J. of Abnormal and Social Psychology 51* (1955), pp. 668-676.
2. Peplau, Hildegard E. "Process and Concept of Learning" in *Some Clinical Approaches to Psychiatric Nursing* (Shirley F. Burd and Margaret A. Marshall, eds.). New York: The Macmillan Co., 1963.

Suggested Readings

Combs, Arthur W., and Snygg, Donald. *Individual Behavior* (rev. ed.). New York: Harper and Bros., 1959.

Peplau, Hildegard E. *Interpersonal Relations in Nursing.* New York: G. P. Putnam's Sons, 1952.

Peplau, Hildegard E. "Themes in Nursing Situations," *Amer. J. Nursing* 53:10 (Oct., 1953), pp. 1221-1223.

Peplau, Hildegard E. "Themes in Nursing Situations," *Amer. J. Nursing* 53:11 (Nov., 1953), pp. 1343-1345.

Peplau, Hildegard E. "Utilizing Themes in Nursing Situations," *Amer. J. Nursing* 54:3 (Mar., 1954), pp. 325-328.

Reik, Theodore. *Listening With the Third Ear.* New York: Farrar, Straus, 1949.

Ujhely, Gertrud B. *The Nurse and Her Problem Patients.* New York: Springer Publishing Co., 1963.

Chapter 8

The Setting, I: Hospital and Long-Term Institution

Nurse and patient do not relate to one another in a vacuum but within the over-all framework of some kind of setting. By virtue of its location, physical setup and purpose and even more, perhaps, by its atmosphere, the setting exerts a powerful influence upon the nurse-patient interaction.

Part of this influence reflects the inherent nature and purpose of the setting. It should be respected by the nurse and serve as a guideline for her actions. Thus, a nurse does not lose sight of the fact that during a home visit she is in someone else's household. She is merely a guest there and has no jurisdiction over the way the hostess runs her affairs. The nurse can make suggestions, of course, but the authority to implement them is not hers.

A setting may also exert noxious influences upon the nurse-patient relationship, however. Its effect may be compared to that of a medication that may bring about side effects quite apart from its intended action and even cause toxicity. Those who are allergic to the medication, have been exposed to it over long periods of time, or have simply had too much of it, may easily become its victim rather than being benefited by it. The nurse needs to be aware of the potential dangers inherent in the setting within which she is interacting with patients, so that she may protect herself and her clients from these dangers or at least apply countermeasures against harm that may already have been done.

In this chapter and the next, we shall highlight some of the effects—both legitimate and noxious—that selected settings may have upon the nurse-patient relationship.

Let us start with the general hospital, the setting in which the majority of nurses are employed. Through its inpatient and out-patient services, the general hospital takes care of emergencies, acute conditions and exacerbations of chronic ones.

The Patient's View of the Hospital Setting

Most patients see the general hospital as a place where they can find help for specific health crises that, for one reason or another, cannot be dealt with adequately at home. These may be minor crises that require only one brief contact with the hospital; for example, a small but profusely bleeding scalp wound. Or, the crisis may require that the patient be hospitalized for a few days while awaiting the completion of a series of diagnostic tests, or following a miscarriage or a tonsillectomy. Such health crises as cardiac infarctions, or certain orthopedic or neurological conditions, may make it necessary for the patient to spend several weeks, or even months, in the hospital.

The duration of the patient's hospital stay is not necessarily related to the severity of his condition. One patient may die soon after his admission to the emergency room, while another may spend many days on the ward following plastic surgery on an unsightly nose.

Whatever the duration of the hospitalization, however, and whatever the outcome of the health crisis in which he finds himself, the patient will rarely consider the general hospital setting to be a substitute for his own home or as a replacement for all other community agencies. It is simply a place where he can get the help he needs so he can go back to his own circumstances, whatever they may be.

The Nurse in the Hospital Setting

The nurse needs to respect this viewpoint on the patient's part and should gear her interaction with him accordingly. That is, in most cases she is there to help him to cope with and, hopefully, overcome a specific health crisis. She is not there to help him solve all the problems he may have, although many nurses and teachers of nurses seem to think so. He may be ill with ulcers that have resulted from the pressures of his job, and the patient may be the first to admit that this is true. Even so, the nurse's immediate responsibility is to assist the patient to deal with what is happening to him *right now* by explaining the various x-ray routines and by helping him to take an active part in the management of his diet. She can be available to him, of course, should he want to talk about his concerns, which, at first, are likely to center around the length of his hospitalization and what this may do to his financial status and to his family. He may fear that his condition is malignant or that he might gain too much weight as a result of his high caloric diet and his physical inactivity.

Similarly, when patients have had a myocardial infarction, the immediate focus of the nurse-patient interaction will be in assisting the patient to integrate the radical change which has taken place in his life by his sudden incapacitation, so that he may be able to make use of the treatment prescribed for him. It may further concern itself with the patient's fears relating to his future, should he wish to discuss these with the nurse.

In fact, if the nurse really concentrates on helping the patient to cope with his current crisis, she has more than enough to do because it involves more than just talking with him. It also involves such concrete actions as making his room bearable to him, if at all possible, selecting roommates for him who will contribute to his well being (and vice versa), putting his bedside table where he can get at it, making sure he has a way of reaching someone on the nursing staff, and being gracious to the patient's visitors and seeing that they have a chair to sit on and at least some degree of privacy during their visit with the patient.

All of these actions on the nurse's part may seem insignificant when compared to the skills required to help him solve his real problems. Yet, what good does the nurse do the patient if she encourages him to open up about his strained relationship with his wife, or about the fact that his son, on whom he dotes so much, is not doing well at college? In pursuing such topics, is she not diverting the patient's energy from his current crisis situation and, therefore, unwittingly being a hindrance to his efforts to cope with it rather than sustaining him in his efforts to meet it?

These questions are not posed to minimize the importance of the patient's problems, nor the fact that they may well have contributed to his current state. Nor are they intended to discount the possibility that the nurse can be quite helpful in assisting him to deal with these problems, either through her own counseling or by referring him to an appropriate person or agency. The point is that now is not the time to do this—not while he is submerged in a crisis.

An objection to this line of reasoning may be based on the fact that the patient, once he is over the crisis and back in his old environment, rarely has the incentive to deal with his problems constructively. Even though this may be quite true, it does not give the nurse license to syphon off energy the patient needs to cope with his imminent situation, simply that he may come to grips with matters of less urgency.

An even more forceful objection may be voiced: "But, look, what happens if you do not help the patient solve the factors that contributed to his illness? Before you know it, he will be back in the hospital, worse than he has ever been before." True, it is often discouraging to the nurse to see patients who have had a short stay at home return to the hospital with the same condition they were treated for during their earlier hospitalization, or a similar one. She feels she has failed the patient in some way. Why put all one's efforts into helping patients get better if, once they are discharged, they go back to their old ways and become ill again?

It seems to me that, because of their deep concern for their patients' welfare, nurses sometimes overestimate the amount of power they really have over the conduct of their patients' lives. Suppose a patient with a leg ulcer that breaks open again and again does come back for the fourth time, because she does not stay off her feet enough. Is this the nurse's fault? Perhaps this woman is the breadwinner for her family and must go to work as a waitress even though she knows she should keep her leg still and elevated on a pillow. Perhaps remaining quiet causes her to start thinking about things that, until now, she has succeeded in keeping out of her awareness. Perhaps she cannot bear to face these thoughts and would rather have a bad leg with all the consequences this may entail. Is it up to the nurse to judge what should be better for the patient in this case? Fortunately, the nurse does not have to make this decision. She is merely asked to help the patient cope with factors pertaining to her readmission. If she and the patient have come to know each other to some degree, the nurse might then inquire into what happened in the woman's life after her last hospitalization. As the talks progress, the nurse might suggest some alternatives of which the patient may not have been aware. She does not press the patient to accept these suggestions, however, she merely asks her to think about them. Perhaps, as a result of these discussions, the patient will be able to deal more effectively with the period following her next discharge. Perhaps not. Such discussions cannot be hurried; they must proceed at the patient's pace, and the patient may be discharged before the nurse has gotten very far with her inquiry.

Working with "abandoned" patients

Sometimes nurses in general hospitals have to work with patients whom physicians have washed their hands of, so to speak. They may be long-term patients who are boarders until a more suitable institution can be found for them. They may be patients whose condition is so far advanced that they cannot be helped by present medical knowledge. The characteristic of both of these kinds of cases is that physicians tend to spend as little time as possible with them and may become annoyed when the nurse asks for guidance concerning their management.

Sensing the physician's lack of interest and sorely missing his direction, the nurse often chafes under this extra burden. She feels rebuffed by the physician and believes that he has abandoned her as well as the patient. No wonder that she sometimes resents the fact that one of these patients has been admitted to her unit. She may say, "What difference does it make if I do take good care of him? No one seems to be interested in what I am doing for him; besides, supposing what I am doing is wrong? What is the use of trying to help him anyway, since before long he will go somewhere else or he will die, regardless of what I do for him?"

What if a particular physician does not care what happens to a certain patient? The nurse has little control over his attitude and feelings. But is it necessary that he appreciate what she does for the patient? Does not this kind of patient need nursing care regardless of his medical prognosis? Why, then, does the nurse ask a medical man questions for which only nurses may have found answers? Would it not be better if she called a group of nurses together, hopefully including some who know a little more than she does, and tried to solve the situation at the nursing level? A plan of action could emerge which, since it would consist of good nursing, would not be medically unsound. Suppose the nurses implement this plan of action and carefully evaluate its results at frequent intervals. After a few days, they may invite the physician to sit in on one of their conferences in order to apprize him of the nursing action taken, not to ask him what they should do. It often happens that as nurses become interested and enthusiastic about a patient, even if only one nurse is involved at first, sooner or later others (including the physician) become interested, too, and their defeatist attitudes change dramatically. The result may be that it is not necessary after all to transfer the patient to a long-term institution. Even if this has to be done, he may have gained enough self-confidence through his experience in the general hospital setting to enable him to approach people in his new environment in such a way that they will react favorably to him. Or, if it happens that the death of a patient cannot be prevented, the nurse will at least have the satisfaction of knowing that she helped to make his last days bearable to him.

Managing the workload

Although the general hospital setting necessitates that the nurse assist the patient to deal with the experience of his immediate crisis, it seems, at the same time, to prevent her from fulfilling this task. The tremendous number of services and activities that go on in a general hospital make it a very busy place indeed. It may take all the energy the nurse has at her disposal to keep up with the workload delegated to her and to deliver the required services on time. That she may then lose sight of the person on whose behalf she struggles, is only too understandable; in fact she may even resent him if his requests or lack of cooperation have taken time which, in her tight schedule, she simply could not spare.

The nurse cannot be blamed for acting the way she does once the pressure of the work has become too much for her; after all, she is only human. As a professional practitioner, however, she must not allow herself to be driven to this point, nor can she merely blame the setting for it and let the matter rest there. She must fight for the survival of her professional focus *before* the impact of the hospital complexity overwhelms her. Even before she accepts a position she may have to question the "powers that be" as to the usual workload of nurses and, in turn, specify how much of that workload she will be able to take on and where she may have to draw the line in order to provide what she considers good nursing care. While employed, she, together with her peers, superiors, and representatives of other disciplines can be instrumental in reorganizing the routines so that the nurses may again have the time they need to give their patients the support to which they are entitled. This is not an easy task, of course, and requires that the nurse have a great deal of administrative knowhow as well as the ability to interpret her point of view to others.

Admittedly, there are some general hospitals where the nurse remains an outsider, an exception to the rule. One can only hope that she will not have to spend her entire working life in such settings.

On the other hand, an increasing number of well-prepared directors of nursing in general hospitals are "going to bat" for the contribution nurses have to offer when given half a chance. As a result, much progress has been made in recent years: Many services now have ward clerks who take care of administrative details; in some hospitals monitoring devices are used to make it possible for nurses to observe several patients at the same time; recently some administrators have been experimenting with having pharmacists dispense routine medications to patients; here and there, the use of computers to streamline the mechanical aspects of nursing care is being investigated. More general hospitals are budgeting salaries for clinical supervisors or advanced nurse-clinicians who serve as role models and resource persons for ward personnel, who work directly with patients and who, in close association with other disciplines, contribute both to the planning and the evaluating of patient care. Doubtless some of these innovations are creating new problems for the nurse. However, as long as she synthesizes her professional focus with the legitimate demands the setting makes on her, she will eventually discover creative ways of solving the problems that arise.

Not all general-hospital patient areas are equally busy. Areas for private patients, for instance, may be very well staffed indeed, with special duty nurses to care for the sickest patients and an ample complement of subprofessional personnel.

This does not mean, however, that these areas are devoid of pitfalls as far as the nurse-patient relationship is concerned. For instance, a nurse may allow herself to be intimidated by a prominent patient's request for privacy—he wants his door closed at all times and does not wish to be disturbed. The nurse hesitates to go into his room to check his progress or his needs, unless she can demonstrate a tangible reason for being there, such as giving a medication, performing a specific procedure or serving his dinner tray. Thus, by obeying the patient's wishes, she may unwittingly neglect his care.

It is by no means easy to establish a relationship with someone who does not wish to be disturbed and who expects little more of a nurse than that she deliver his medicine on time and perform other basic nursing functions.

Is it necessary, however, that the nurse convince him of her worth and many-sidedness before she can give him the nursing care to which he is entitled? What does it matter if he has less need to confide in the nurse than patients with fewer financial, intellectual and community resources? He may have a long-standing relationship of mutual trust and respect with his physician who, therefore, communicates openly and honestly with him. In that case, there may be little or no need for the nurse to interpret hospital routines to the patient or to correct any misapprehensions he may have, except, of course, for the business of the closed door. Perhaps the nurse will need to ask the physician to explain to the patient the need for her frequent observational visits to his room. Perhaps she, herself, can tactfully explain the reasons for these visits, especially if she demonstrates good judgment by being skillful, reliable and thoughtful in her care of the patient. Perhaps the need for her entering his room at frequent intervals should have been explained to him immediately after he was admitted.

Avoiding regimentation

Wards with rows and rows of beds containing indigent patients may present the nurse with problems diametrically opposite to those encountered in private-room areas. Instead of being intimidated by the fact of each patient's individuality, she may tend to lose sight of it altogether. She does not set out to do this, of course. She merely reacts as anyone would when asked to deal with a large group of people at the same time: She perceives them as a mass, one entity, and not as an aggregate of individuals. This perception is even more pronounced if she has relatively little in common with the group, i.e., if its members are less successful economically than she is, less well educated—particularly in health matters—and if their habits and beliefs differ considerably from her own.

Unless the nurse checks herself somewhere along the line, she will be tempted to act in accordance with her perception. Since she has lost sight of the individual, she may consider the aggregate with which she has to deal as an inferior mass, incapable of self-regulation and which, therefore, needs to be regimented into some semblance of order. Anyone who falls out of step is seen as potentially dangerous, for he may promote disorder which could easily lead to a state of chaos.

How many of us have not, at one time or another, acted in one or more of the following ways: turned off the lights in the ward at a certain hour because it was "bedtime" regardless of whether one of the patients still had to get undressed, or whether another one wanted to finish reading the last paragraph in his paper; told a ward patient who requested that we refill his water pitcher to wait because soon everyone would receive clean pitchers of fresh ice-water; wakened women on the maternity ward at three-thirty in the morning with the clanking of bedpans and warned the patient who refused to make use of this routine that she had better not ask for a bedpan later while the other women would be nursing their babies; started giving morning care at one end of the ward and systematically worked our way through to the other end, regardless of which patients might have been in most urgent need of being bathed and changed; told a clinic patient who inquired at the nurses' station how much longer he would have to wait, to go back to his bench and sit down, that when his turn came his name would be called just like all the other names.

Unless we build strong safeguards into our work when caring for large numbers of patients, we will succumb to this kind of regimentation. One such safeguard might be to mentally break up the large ward into small segments or units of not more than ten people. If at all possible, one staff member should be in charge of each of these units. If there are not enough nurses for this kind of staffing, the head nurse can at least keep these demarcations in mind while observing the patients and planning for their care. She may ask herself: "Who in unit one is the sickest patient?" "What do I know about the patients who comprise unit two?" "Can the patients in unit four wait for their care until those in the other three units have been cared for?"

Another safeguard against regimenting one's patients may be to know a great deal about the group to which, by virtue of their various characteristics, they belong. Let me explain. Suppose a nurse works on a ward of paraplegic male patients in a Federal institution. The men come from all walks of life and from a variety of ethnic and religious backgrounds. Some are young and some are middle aged; some are married or divorced, others single. Now, the nurse who is willing to look for it, can find a great deal of information in the literature about how men tend to react to being paralyzed. Do differences in age cause differences in this reaction? How do men from different backgrounds vary in their reactions to such illnesses? How might paralyzed men feel about their futures as males and how do these feelings get translated into their interactions with women, especially their wives?

If the nurse knows what to look for, the formless crowd in front of her will give way to a kaleidoscope of patterns. Not only will she recognize the phenomena she has learned about from the literature, but she will also notice variations within these phenomena, and even in the patients' behavior, which might be radically different from what she had expected. Because she understands what she is seeing, and because what she is seeing has developed a great deal of meaning for her, the nurse becomes more and more appreciative of what she sees. She begins to recognize and like every patient on the ward as an individual in his own right, and no longer has any need to resort to coercive measures.

This is to be expected, for when one takes a great deal of

trouble to learn about a certain subject, one develops, at the same time, a capacity to appreciate its individual manifestations. The layman who drinks a glass of wine may not be able to distinguish between those characteristics which are common to all wines and those which make the color, flavor and consistency of this particular wine especially appealing. Only the person who knows dogs appreciates the "dogness" of his poodle while at the same time enjoying those characteristics that are uniquely his.

Themes in General Hospital Services

The nurse in the general hospital setting needs to be alert to the fact that each hospital service is permeated by an atmosphere containing one or more characteristic themes. These themes might be identical for staff and patients, or different for each group. For instance, the theme binding the emergency-room staff together might be that of quick and efficient action, while the theme of patients and their families is often one of shock and bewilderment. The contradiction between these two themes is not necessarily noxious. What better remedy is there for someone who is baffled and perhaps still stunned by a sudden, unexpected injury, than to come into the hands of a physician and a nurse who both know exactly what to do and who work carefully and efficiently. The nurse must watch out, however, that she does not get carried away with her own theme to the extent that it drowns out those of her clients. She needs to be attuned to their themes and relate to them accordingly; that is, while she will be very clear and concrete in her communications with the patient and the persons who may have accompanied him to the hospital, she will in no way allow the swiftness and purposefulness of her movements to be diminished. She will give them only one or two directions at a time, for she knows one cannot be expected to remember more than this while one's anxiety level is high. Thus, she will not direct them to the x-ray department by telling them to go straight to the center light, then turn left and once more to the right. Instead, she will send someone with the patient and inform his relatives that he is going to be x-rayed now to find out if any bones are broken and that the physician will see them in the emergency room soon after the pictures have been taken.

On some services, such as a ward for patients with eye diseases, the theme for most staff members may be routine care—drops every hour, hot applications, aspirin for pain, and feeding patients who have bandages over both eyes. Yet, it is no routine matter for a person to undergo a cataract operation, for example. It is a strange experience to suddenly not be able to see, because one's eyes are covered with bandages. It is anything but routine to have to lie still on one's back, especially at night. The patient may be afraid to go to sleep for fear he will turn over without knowing it and thus, through his own doing, lose his sight. It would seem that by keeping in mind the importance which eyes and sight have for a person, the nurse could easily refrain from being too matter-of-fact in her attitude.

The theme on an obstetric ward, as far as staff members and some patients are concerned, may be one of cheerfulness and hope. This is understandable, for what greater joy is there than participating in the thrilling event of birth? Yet, for many women about to become mothers, there is nothing thrilling or cheerful about having to go through labor. Nor is a 16-year-old, unwed girl likely to feel particularly cheerful over the prospect of giving her child over to an adoption agency. Thus, the theme of cheerfulness may sometimes be inappropriate. The nurse may be able to counteract an inappropriate prevailing atmosphere and help to replace it by one of understanding, if those working with her are willing to follow her example. Even when her co-workers do not cooperate, she can still avoid being affected by their attitudes and remain human and understanding on her own. To maintain an attitude which runs counter to the prevailing one is not an easy task, however. It creates a certain amount of tension and disharmony (i.e., cognitive imbalance) in oneself, in the others with whom one differs, and in one's relationships with them. It will be up to the individual nurse to decide whether she can endure the strain and still act in accordance with the theme she thinks is right for the particular situation; whether she should look for another, more congenial work setting; or whether, to meet her own need for belonging, she should finally give in to the pressure of the atmosphere surrounding her.

Effects of the Long-Term Setting on the Relationship

Let us now look at the way in which such long-term settings as chronic disease hospitals, homes for the retarded, state mental institutions and nursing homes may affect the relationship between nurse and patient. The characteristic nature of all of these settings is that they can keep most of their patients, or residents, as they sometimes call them, for a much longer time than the general hospital can. Even though there has been a trend in recent years to rehabilitate the chronically ill and disabled, and to reincorporate them into the community, all long-term institutions harbor a large number of persons who may never again return to the community. Thus, in contrast to the general hospital setting, such an institution is likely to become "home," or at least a second home, to many patients. Therefore, the thoughtful nurse will do everything in her power to make the atmosphere of the setting as homelike as possible. This implies also that, although she provides the necessary nursing care, her interaction with her patients will center more on matters of daily living than on the patients' diseases or the handicaps that may have occurred as a result of them.

It is not always easy to keep nurse-patient relationships centered on matters of daily living, however. First, many patients in long-term institutions have not yet reached that stage of acceptance of their condition that would enable them to "make the best of it." Second, since they are likely to associate a nurse with illness, they may tend to relate to her on the basis of their symptoms rather than as one person to another. They are even willing, on occasion, to manufacture new complaints lest the nurse be bored with their usual symptomatology. Third, nurses might unwittingly go along with this deception, for they may feel more secure in their ability to help patients with their physical complaints than with other aspects of their lives. Finally, the organizational structure of the setting may be such that it would be extremely difficult for the nurse, if not altogether impossible, to provide a homelike atmosphere.

The patient's acceptance of his condition

As to the first difficulty—the patient's reluctance to accept his condition—this phenomenon is found in an almost unbelievably large number of patients in long-term disease hospitals and homes for the aged and chronically infirm. It is usually the result of the patient's having remained stuck, as it were, in a certain stage of grief over the loss he has incurred by virtue of his condition. Whether this loss is a material one or symbolic in nature does not actually matter; it is real enough to him.

One may ask, "But why can the patient not resolve his grief? Why can he not negotiate one stage of it after another until he finally reaches a stage at which he can accept his loss?" Well, he simply may not have the power to do it alone, and perhaps no one has been very helpful to him in the matter. Usually, however, the actual situation is quite the opposite. Well-meaning health practitioners, and the patient's family and friends, eager to see him rehabilitated, may have tried to push him along too fast, rather than simply offering him support when he needed it. Perhaps, also, his present loss has opened a floodgate of memories of other serious losses he may have sustained previously and which, due to his upbringing or the circumstances that prevailed, he may not have had the chance to integrate by suffering through them. Instead, he may have pushed them out of his awareness so that he could take on new responsibilities that he did not necessarily want and which frequently were premature for his level of development. Now he reflects on these incidents and mourns not only his present loss, but also all those that he could not permit himself to mourn at the times they occurred.

No wonder, then, that the nurse may find him breaking all the rules of the institution, since he may still need to deny his present condition. No wonder that he may bemoan his misfortune day in, day out, and that the nurse finds it impossible to engage him in activities which she knows could bring him at least some pleasure. No wonder, further, that staff and patients alike may be very much upset about his querulousness and that no one wants to spend time with him, for it may be easier for him to pick fights with people than to blame fate for the injustices he feels it has handed him.

What are the implications of this protracted grief for the nurse's interaction with her patient? I would suggest that she set the focus for the interaction on as *broad* a base as possible and that she allow the patient all the time he needs to talk about his various losses, regardless of whether he may wish to start with his present one or with one which happened many years ago. At first, she might do this best by encouraging the patient to tell her about *himself*. Then, whenever she has an opportunity to spend some time with him, she can suggest that he tell her more about the topic on which he has embarked. He may need to go over one or another episode repeatedly. This is all right; there is no need to hurry him. After all, he is bringing up a lifetime's worth of pent-up emotion and unresolved suffering. As he gradually releases the feelings he has held in check for such a long time, the patient may feel as if he has been relieved of a tremendous burden. As a result, he may be enabled to move along on the path leading to the acceptance of his current loss.

The nurse will have to let the other members of her staff know what she is trying to do to help the patient. This way, they are prepared for the possibility that the formerly mischievous and uncooperative patient may become mopey and feel sorry for himself; that the apathetic and depressed patient may suddenly become querulous and find fault with the food, the temperature of his bath water and the way he is being lifted into his chair; and that the patient who has been so disagreeable to everyone that patients and staff avoided him whenever they could, suddenly asks for permission to participate in rehabilitative group activities. The nurse must also help other staff members not to hold the patient's past behavior against him, so that his transition into the next stage of his grief will not be hampered by their attitudes.

I believe firmly that, given such an opportunity to talk, the patient is very likely to uncover inner resources which he had been unable to tap before and that will serve, eventually, to help him find a way of life which, although different from that of his past, may still be meaningful to him.

The patient's need to produce symptoms

Some patients seem to find it hard to conceive that the nurse would be interested in them if they are not in physical distress. This may be illustrated by the fact that, in the absence of real symptoms, such patients may be inclined to invent one or another symptom, just to make sure the busy nurse devotes some of her time to them. However, since the purpose of the long-term institution is to help patients make some use of their lives in spite of their handicaps, it would be foolhardy for the nurse to fall into the trap the patient has, in all innocence, laid out for her. It is better for her to focus, *literally,* on the "patient as a person" right from the start of their relationship, instead of treating him as someone suffering from a disease. This does not mean that she is excused from doing all that is necessary—and everything in her power—to slow up the disease process and reduce the handicap, but only that she not make the patient's disease process the pivot around which her interaction with him revolves. It should be peripheral to the fact that he is a person who has lived a life before he came into her care and may still have a number of interests which are related to his past. That is, in addition to inquiring into the patient's life and losses, the nurse should also inquire into his interests and then, for example, remind him of a baseball game on television and follow this up the next day by asking him what he thought of it. She might bring in newspaper clippings and magazines that could be of interest to him. She could make sure that he is aware of institutional outings which he might like to join.

It helps, of course, if the nurse happens to have the same interests as her patient even though, in sports, for example, her allegiance might be with an opposing team. The resulting, hopefully humorous, bickering betwen them might prove most stimulating to the patient. If the nurse does not share any of the patient's interests, she can at least see that he has the company of someone who does, and she can inquire every so often how the patient and his partner are getting along.

Obstacles to acquiring new skills

The third reason why it may be difficult for the nurse to assist patients to acquire new skills in living may be her reluctance to focus on these skills rather than on the patients' pathology. This is quite understandable, since nurses have rarely had opportunity for practice in this area during the course of their basic nursing education. It is supposed, perhaps rightly, that a nurse knows how to lead the life of an average person with all the ramifications this might entail, such as going shopping, taking buses, or taking a car to a garage to be repaired. It is also supposed, with less justification perhaps, that there is nothing difficult about imparting such skills to one's patients, should this be necessary. Yet, unless one is conscious of what one is doing and unless one knows how to make the action explicit to another person, one may find it hard to teach simple skills of living. Also, unless the nurse has thought about it beforehand, it may seem strange to her that a patient who is permitted to go out and buy a dress would rather have the nurse do it for her than choose one herself. Yet, the patient, whose movements and ability to speak are considerably slowed down as a result of her condition, may be terrified of city noises and hustling crowds which seem to want to drag her along with them or push her to the ground. She may be afraid that the driver and the passengers will ridicule her or be rude to her if she cannot step on or off the bus fast enough to suit them. She may be worried that, because of her speech handicap, she will not be able to state her business clearly and that the saleslady might become impatient with her and rebuff her in front of the other customers. She may be afraid that she will not find a bathroom as frequently as she might need to use one.

Well, then, why doesn't the nurse go shopping with the patient? She could give support wherever it is needed; she could intervene tactfully, when necessary, and thus spare the patient some of the embarrassment she dreads.

"Yes, but is this nursing?" one may ask, and "Where do you plan to draw the line?" Well, if nursing has to do with sustaining patients in their experience how better can the nurse sustain a patient who has been isolated from the world for a long time than by orienting her as to what she might expect to experience on her first shopping trip; to rehearse with her some of the steps she will be taking; to go with her the first two or three times so that the impact of the outer world will not be too overwhelming for her; and to assist her, if necessary, to find a dress she will like and that she can afford?

The nurse may wonder who has time for such extra services to patients. Yet, is this an "extra" service to a patient who, by virtue of her condition and the waning interest of her family and friends, may have lost touch with the community? Is it not of vital importance to her, even if she will never go home again, to keep her contact with the outer world alive for as long as this is possible?

Besides, who else but the nurse, as a qualified practitioner should have the right to decide which activities will be included in her work schedule? Of course, she will not spend several hours with one patient on such a shopping trip unless this seems to her to be an important aspect of the patient's care, and unless the unit is adequately staffed. If it is not necessary that a person highly skilled in the art of sustaining patients accompany her, she will certainly either let the patient go alone or send someone along whose time is less costly to the institution than her own.

Influence of the power structure of the institution

Finally, the fourth condition that may make it difficult for the nurse to help patients to reestablish some kind of meaningful life for themselves is the power structure of the institution. Unfortunately, many long-term settings seem to attract personnel who prefer security to risk-taking, and a rigid system of rules to individual responsibility. They would rather "pass the buck" to their superiors than "stick their necks out" for what they believe in. This kind of behavior may have certain advantages for the staff, because it keeps them from getting unduly involved with their patients and thus they can save their energies for activities outside the sphere of their work. It is not advantageous to the patient, however, because in this kind of hierarchical system, he is unfailingly placed at the bottom of the hierarchy.

The reasons for this phenomenon are many (and may not all hold true in all cases). One of the chief reasons is that the patient's physical or emotional condition has rendered him defenseless. Also, he does not usually enjoy the same kind of community support as does his colleague in the general hospital. In many instances, the patient's family has—by and large—turned him over to the institution. Although they may come to visit him and even take him home for weekends and holidays, they have had to abdicate the main responsibility for his care. Regardless of whether they feel pleased or guilty about having done this, they may not feel free to complain about the care the patient is getting or the way he is treated by the personnel, for they may have reason to fear that the staff member in question, if reprimanded, might retaliate by treating the patient even worse than before.

A third reason for the patient's being at the bottom of the institution's hierarchy may be the fact that he operates alone, as it were, without the support of his peers. He may never have possessed the ability to establish peer relationships; he may mistrust the other patients or be afraid of them because of their illnesses; or he may have become demoralized by the pressures of the institution. In any case, he is unable to pool the resources of his fellow patients into some kind of power system which might help him to voice some opposition to his status or the quality of his care.

It is true that there has recently been enacted a considerable amount of legislation that is aimed at safeguarding the patient's rights in some categories of long-term institutions. Responsible administrators are also making efforts to strengthen patients' social standing through such means as patient-government organizations. Most directors of nursing investigate any report of cruelty on the part of staff members—if they receive such reports—and dismiss the person in question, if evidence is found that the complaint is true. These are hopeful signs indeed. Yet, in many long-term institutions these measures do not amount to more than token gestures which do not really alter the basic order of the hierarchy. Consequently, everyone except the patient continues to take orders from above and to give orders to those who are below him. Because of his position in the hierarchical structure, the patient may only *take* orders, for there is no one below him to give orders to. Also, everyone else in the hierarchy can make decisions that pertain to his own sphere of authority. Everyone, that is, except the patient. He has no authority whatever. Others decide for him when he is to get up, bathe and shave, what clothes he should wear, what he should eat and, sometimes, even when he should use the toilet.

As we have seen earlier in this chapter, some of this kind of regimentation is also found in the general hospital setting. The difference is that the patient in that setting is subjected to such regimentation for a relatively short time and, knowing this, he can usually put up with it without losing too much self-esteem; he may even be able to laugh about it and forget it, once he has gone home. However, since the long-term institution *is* the patient's home, one may well wonder what it does to a person to be continuously denied a choice in practically every area of his daily life. Is not the integrity and uniqueness of personality based on a repetition of individual choices? This is the crux of the matter, for after a while, the patient's personality, his uniqueness, tends to disintegrate. He becomes apathetic and more and more detached from his surroundings until, finally, he merely vegetates in a kind of semiconscious twilight state.

Of course, not all patients give in to the system. Some will fight for their independence and become trouble-makers. Others may circumvent the hospital system and obtain self-confirmation by devious means. They may steal money from their neighbors, or they may go out to the street corner and beg and then buy liquor with the proceeds and have a party with their wardmates at night while the staff is dozing. Other patients may succeed in becoming the hospital workers' pet, simply because they are likeable, or because they do some of the workers' more unpleasant tasks for them. These patients usually enjoy extra privileges which, if not necessarily therapeutic for them in the long run, at least raise them above the lowest level in the hierarchy.

The picture painted here may seem rather grim and perhaps exaggerated. However, if one takes the trouble to look around or to read the descriptions that such well-known authors as Goffman (1), Belknap (2), Greenblatt and his colleagues (3), and others (4, 5) have given of some long-term institutions, one will have to admit that this account of the power structure in many of these institutions is not invented.

What, then, is the nurse who wishes to change the situation in such an institution to do? Beat her head against the wall? Or pound against it with her bare knuckles? No, she should not do anything of this sort, but she certainly should be very much aware of what she is getting into if she decides to work in a long-term institution of the type just described. If she is an innovator who likes to be able to see great changes actually take place before her eyes, she had best take a very careful look at both the medical director of the institution and the director of nursing. Are they really interested in changing things for the better? Are they willing to sacrifice some of their power by promoting a gradual decentralization of the institutional framework with a consequent loosening up of the strict hierarchy? Or are they merely giving lip service to the idea of such change? The nurse might find the answers to these questions, before she accepts employment, if she has an opportunity to go on the wards and spend some time observing the kind of interaction that takes place between the supervisor and her staff and between staff members and their patients, as well as that which takes place among staff members themselves. Does the nurse on the ward call the practical nurse to give a glass of water to a patient? Does the practical nurse merely stand with her hands behind her back and wait for the aide to take a rectal temperature and then ask the aide to clean the thermometer and hand it over to her, so that she may read it and record the reading on the chart? Does the aide call a "working patient" to mop the floor if one of the patients has failed to reach the bathroom in time?

It is not enough, by the way, for the chief physician *or* the chief nurse to be progressive. To achieve change, *both* must work in the same direction, otherwise only the one who is able to block the other's efforts will succeed. Again, the nurse can learn a great deal about what goes on between these two from observing interactions at the ward level, for attitudes have a way of transmitting themselves from the upper to the lower echelons. What happens during rounds, for instance? Is the physician interested in what the head nurse has to contribute, or does he brush off her comments with some non-committal mumbo jumbo and proceed to the next patient? Does he have to ask nurses repeatedly not to speak for the patient but to let him speak for himself? Or does the physician prefer that the nursing staff shield him from the patient's problems so that he can write his orders in peace and go on to the next four wards which are also under his care?

Of course, not every nurse is an innovator. Besides, even an innovator might do well to work within static settings occasionally in order to see what she might be able to do to effect change. She would have to set her goals accordingly, however, and not try to fight the system with her superior knowledge; this could only result in ridicule and heartache and an utter waste of her energies. Instead, she might remind herself of the central concern of her profession and use it as the guideline for her work. The fact that the patients are in this particular setting is a reality that she did nothing to bring about. She can, however, by judicious nursing, sustain her patients in their experience of the "total institution" in which they happen to be confined. She may not be able to do a great deal to help patients make their own decisions as far as the ward routine is concerned, for the combined power of the ward staff may be far greater than her own. Even so, there is still a great deal she can do for those patients with whom she comes into contact. She can help them to learn that, no matter what the power structure in the situation, other people can control them only up to a certain point, because it is still within the patient's power to choose the way he will accept his situation. Even though he may have to take his shower together with five other patients, it is up to him whether he will let himself be humiliated by this procedure. He is free to think whatever he pleases about those who submit him to this humiliation, although it may not be to his advantage to say it aloud. If he looks hard enough he may find little things on the ward that he can feel free to enjoy regardless of the way he is being treated—a brief chat with his neighbor, a concert transmitted on his little radio, a magazine article or a patch of sunshine on the porch.

How often the nurse will be successful in helping patients rise above the system will depend to a large extent on her ability to mobilize the patient's inner resources, provided, of course, that he has such resources; but the chances are that she will be able to provide solace for many a patient who would otherwise have been disconsolate.

It is hoped that concurrently with sustaining the patient in his experience, the nurse will be able to exert some influence on the staff. Thus, through informal conferences, she might give them opportunities to think and talk about their ideas of what the patients' experiences on their wards might be like. As this line of investigation is opened to them, staff members may come to realize that many hardships and humiliations that they are (unwittingly, I am sure) imposing on patients need not occur. Before long, they may come up with suggestions for providing better care which, since they thought of them themselves, are more likely to be implemented and followed than if they had been requested by the nurse.

Effects of the setting on patients' and nurses' themes

The most prevalent themes one encounters in patients in long-term institutions are those of loss, abandonment and apathy, while those most evident in the staff members are indifference, false hope and hopelessness.

The themes of loss and apathy have been discussed in the preceding pages. As to abandonment, this, too, is a difficult theme for the nurse to handle. Although it may be a very painful experience indeed for any person to enter a long-term institution, it is an even more painful experience for a patient to realize that his family members, after visiting him less and less frequently, have finally stopped coming in at all. They don't come even on holidays, or on the patient's birthday, or—and this is the greatest blow of all—on the occasion of his only daughter's marriage. There may be many reasons for the family members' need to increase distance between themselves and the patient. They may feel guilty about what they have done to him, even though it was the only thing they could have done and still be fair to everyone concerned, including the patient. To regain their family stability, they may have had to close ranks after his departure and, as a result, their concern for him has perhaps become more peripheral than it used to be. They may be tired of his pleading that they visit him more often and of his accusations that they do not come often enough. To avoid having to make excuses for not coming, they may come even less often than before.

Nurses are often disturbed by the way a patient's family seems to abandon him to the institution. They may have definite ideas as to the responsibilities of families toward their sick members and may take it very much to heart if their patients' families do not live up to these ideas. The result is that they tend to react in one or another of the following ways: They may try to cover up for the delinquent family by making excuses for them, because they feel that this will help the patient to maintain his trust in his relatives; or they may encourage the patient to contact the family by mail or telephone and to let them know that he misses them and would very much like to see them. The nurse may contact a family member herself, or, when one of the family does come to see the patient, reprimand him for not taking more interest in his relative.

Unfortunately, these nurses do not seem to realize that by their meddling they may be putting added pressure on the family and thus may achieve results which are the exact opposite of those they are trying to achieve.

Wouldn't it be better for the nurse to spend her efforts in helping the patient to see and gradually accept his situation as it really is? If, in her eyes, the family behaves in a shameful way, does this shame necessarily fall on the patient? Does the fact that his family abandons him make him any less worthy a person? Is he not also an individual, besides being a member of a family? The nurse who is convinced of the patient's dignity as a person in his own right will find ways of gradually helping him to make better use of his energy than wasting it on the illusion that his family will soon reincorporate him into their midst. She may also be able to help him learn not to waste his energy in futile resentment, but rather to use it for the purpose of creating a life for himself under the existing circumstances. In time, he will develop a certain degree of independence from his family members. Then, if they do come to see him, he may genuinely enjoy their visits, while at the same time being able to let them stay away.

As to the staff's theme of indifference, it is hoped that the nurse herself will be able to demonstrate a more positive example. It is hoped, also, that it will be within her power to provide opportunities for staff members to share with her their experiences and suggestions concerning patient care.

The theme of hopelessness is a very dangerous theme indeed. Not only does it paralyze the staff's ability to give creative care, but it is also likely to spread to the patients and cause their outlook on life to be even more gloomy than it may already be. Hopelessness is really a way of defending oneself against feeling helpless (6), and helplessness occurs when one lets one's inability to function in one area spread to all other areas of functioning, even though these other areas are perfectly intact.

The head nurse who understands the themes of hopelessness and helplessness may be able to assist her staff to overcome them. Instead of letting them talk at great length about their discouragements, she can direct the discussion toward the areas in which they are legitimately helpless. It may take some time to find these areas, since the staff members, although aware of their being discouraged, may not know the reason for it. Eventually, though, they will express what really bothers them: No matter how good the care they give to their patients and no matter how hard they try, sooner or later their patients' health begins to decline until, finally, there is nothing anyone can do for them. This is true, of course, since a large number of patients in long-term institutions suffer from conditions that are degenerative in nature.

Once the head nurse has helped her staff to identify the areas in which they are really helpless, (for example, their inability to bring patients suffering from degenerative diseases back to health), she can explore with them those areas of service in which they can still be of considerable use to their patients. Finally, she can help her staff to accept those limitations that they cannot alter and to apply themselves to those areas of care that do lie within their own areas of responsibility. After a while, feelings of hopelessness will give way to feelings of satisfaction, for instead of chafing against the inevitable, the nursing staff will concentrate on providing the care that their patients deserve.

It is not enough to discuss this matter once with one's staff members, however, for the theme of hopelessness may reemerge each time a patient to whom the staff has become particularly attached, suddenly takes a turn for the worse. The nurse will have to direct her staff's attention to this theme frequently during ward conferences or while working beside one or another member of her team.

Sometimes the nurse will find that her staff is exuding the theme of false hope so as not to appear to feel hopeless. That is, the nursing personnel act as if the actuality of the patient's condition did not exist, as if the patient were not failing, as if everything would soon be all right. The chances are that they need to express this theme in order to survive. In other words, instead of resorting to hopelessness, they are using false hope as a defense against feeling utterly helpless. The effect of this attitude on the patients, though different, is equally bad, for patients know better than to take staff members' hopefulness at face value. They take it for the defense against the truth which it really is and may, as a result, feel even more isolated in their condition than they ever had before.

Once the nurse has established a relationship with her ward staff, she may, at an opportune moment, have to confront them with their unwarranted cheerfulness. If she allows time for them to reply to her confrontation, she will soon be able to get at the underlying themes of hopelessness and helplessness and then assist her staff to cope with these.

References

1. Goffman, Erving. *Asylums*. Chicago: Aldine Publishing Co., 1962.
2. Belknap, Ivan. *Human Problems of a State Mental Hospital*. New York: McGraw-Hill Book Co., 1956.
3. Greenblatt, Milton *et al. From Custodial to Therapeutic Patient Care*. New York: Russell Sage Foundation, 1955.
4. Caudill, William A. *The Psychiatric Hospital as a Small Society*. Cambridge, Mass.: Harvard University Press, 1958.

5. Von Mering, Otto, and King, Stanley. *Remotivating the Mental Patient*. New York: Russell Sage Foundation, 1957.
6. Ujhely, Gertrud B. *The Nurse and Her Problem Patients*. New York: Springer Publishing Co., 1963.

Suggested Readings

Bettelheim, Bruno. *The Informed Heart: Autonomy in a Mass Age*. Glencoe, Ill.: The Free Press, 1960.

Blumberg, Jeanne E., and Drummond, Eleanor E. *Nursing Care of the Long-Term Patient*. New York: Springer Publishing Co., 1963.

Brown, Esther Lucile. *Newer Dimensions of Patient Care*. New York: Russell Sage Foundation. Part I, 1961; Part II, 1962; Part III, 1964.

Cantril, Hadley. *The "Why" of Man's Experience*. New York: The Macmillan Co., 1950.

Coser, Rose Laub. *Life in the Ward*. East Lansing, Mich.: Michigan State University Press, 1962.

Frankl, Viktor E. *Man's Search for Meaning*. Boston: Beacon Press, 1963.

Heider, Fritz. *The Psychology of Interpersonal Relations*. New York: John Wiley & Sons, 1958.

Rauffenhart, Mary. "Drug Administration by Automation," *Nursing Clinics of North America 1*:4 (Dec., 1966), pp. 611-620.

Rosenberg, Mervin, and Carriker, Delores. "Automating Nurses Notes," *American Journal of Nursing 66*:5 (May, 1966), pp. 1021-1023.

Rouslin, Sheila. "Chronic Helpfulness: Maintenance or Intervention," *Perspectives in Psychiatric Care 1*:1 (Jan.-Feb., 1963), pp. 25-28.

Smith, Dorothy W., and Gips, Claudia D. *Care of the Adult Patient* (2nd ed.). Philadelphia: J. B. Lippincott Co., 1966.

Thaler, Otto F. "Grief and Depression," *Nursing Forum* 5:2 (1966), pp. 8-22.

Ujhely, Gertrud B. "Grief and Depression—Implications for Preventive and Therapeutic Nursing Care," *Nursing Forum* 5:2 (1966), pp. 23-35.

Weil, T. P., and Weil, J. W. "The Use of Computer Systems in Patient Care," *Nursing Forum* 6:2 (1967), pp. 207 ff.

Chapter 9

The Setting, II: The Patient's Home

One obvious difference between the patient's home environment and the hospital or long-term institution is that the basic purpose of the institution is to give care to sick people. Its activities, whether carried out well or poorly, are centered on this purpose and geared to its fulfillment. In one's home, however, illness is the exception rather than the rule. Consequently, the nurse who works in the home setting is likely to have to improvise a great deal in order to provide patient care in the existing environment.

This is much easier said than done. When working in the institution, the nurse has quite a bit of control over the patient's routines and activities and also over his environment, but in the patient's home it is the family who is in control. The professional worker remains an outsider—at worst, an intruder, at best, a welcome guest.

To adjust to this difference in her status, the nurse may need to change her entire perspective with relation to the patient and his family. In the institutional setting she tends to see her main responsibility as centering on her patient and she is only peripherally concerned with his family members whom she considers as not always welcome adjuncts of the patient. In the home setting, on the other hand, the nurse usually deals with an entire family of which at least one member happens to be in need of health counseling or nursing care.

As long as she continues to act in the capacity of a private-duty or visiting nurse rendering direct care to the sick family member, the differences between the settings may not be too apparent. The chances are that she will retain a great deal of authority over the patient's immediate environment and that she will receive the full cooperation of the family. When the private-duty nurse leaves the bedside, however, lines of authority and role relationships are likely to become less clear. Suppose, for instance, that she would like to have some fruit juice for her patient who, by the way, may safely be left alone for the time it would take for her to fetch it. By getting the juice herself, is she apt to enter territory that is "out of bounds" for her—territory ruled by a cook or maid, or even by the lady of the house? On the other hand, if she asks that the juice be brought to the patient's room, will an indignant household staff consider her presumptuous, lazy, or perhaps both?

Where is the private-duty nurse supposed to go while the family members visit the patient? Where is she to have her meals? In the patient's room? In the dining room together with the family? In the kitchen with the household staff? Or off somewhere by herself? How do her expectations in this respect coincide with those of the other members of the household?

The answers to these ticklish questions depend partly upon the situation in which the nurse finds herself and partly on her own personality. Some nurses are endowed with a great deal of tact and can fit easily into any setting without losing sight of their main goals. Others may find it very difficult to exhibit social graces while in the role of a professional nurse. Trying hard to be sociable, they may bore the family with long accounts of other cases they have had or of their vacations between cases. By trying too hard to impress the family with what a professional nurse does and does not do, they may create more work for the members of the household than there would have been without a nurse. Other nurses may be too eager to make themselves useful, and may tend to usurp the functions of other persons in the home. This may result not only in a profound feeling of helplessness in these others, but also in neglect of the nurse's own responsibilities.

Private-duty nursing in the home setting is very difficult to carry out and should not be attempted by nurses who are too conscious of their professional prestige, or by those who have little tolerance for ambiguity in regard to their functions or their status in the family.

When the patient who is receiving nursing care at home has improved sufficiently to dispense with his private-duty nurse, or when it becomes apparent that his condition is likely to remain stationary for a long period of time, private-duty nursing usually ends and visiting nursing begins. The visiting nurse is then faced with making a decision about whom she should entrust with the responsibility for the patient's care. Will it be the person who has demonstrated the greatest interest and skill? The person who heads up the family? Or the person with whom the nurse has found it easiest to communicate?

Importance of Identifying the Family Leader

Actually, it is not up to the visiting nurse to decide which member of the household will take care of the patient. This decision should be made by the family and is usually reached, or at least strongly influenced, by the most powerful person in the group. The nurse will probably have formed some idea as to the identity of this most powerful person, however, and it is her responsibility to sustain and encourage this person so that he may use his power to the patient's best advantage.

Such action may be self-evident if the key person is the head of the household and if his use of power consists of lending support and strength to the others so that they all may be better able to cope with the crisis.

Sometimes, however, the most powerful person happens to be a junior member of the family or even the patient himself. What then? Would it not create an awkward situation if the nominal head were left out of the deliberations? There is no reason why the nurse cannot include in her planning the person nominally in charge of family affairs as well as the one who really holds the reins. Also, there is really no reason why the patient himself, if at all able to do so, should not be given a voice in making the decisions which have to do with his own care.

What if the most powerful person in the family, instead of using his strength for the benefit of all concerned; tends to dominate and to intimidate these others, perhaps in an attempt to conceal from them his own lack of ability? Wouldn't it be better in such a case to defend the weaker members of the household, especially the patient, against this person's noxious influence?

What happens when the nurse allies herself with the intimidated ones? The chances are that this will represent a threat to the person who has been in control, or at least it will antagonize him. Further, in order to reinforce his position, he will be likely to apply more severe countermeasures, one of which might well consist of barring the nurse from further entry into his home.

Would it not be better for everyone concerned if the nurse, without judging such a person or his actions, were to listen sympathetically to his account of what his current situation means to him? Her understanding attitude may convey to him that his difficulty in coping with the events in his home is indeed realistic. This, in turn, may help him to regain a certain degree of security and feeling of self worth. As a result, he may not feel as much need to prove himself by bullying the other members of his family as he did before, and hence may gradually relax his control over them. In fact, having had this opportunity to be considered a person in his own right may well open up the possibility that he will accord the same privilege to others in the family.

Of course, the nurse's chances for success are greater if these negative power operations have been a means of trying to cope with the stress of a sudden crisis for which the family was totally unprepared. In many instances, however, domination of all family members by one of them is a way of life rather than a response to an emergency. In such cases, the nurse must not expect to see a great deal of change as a result of her intervention, for the one who wields the power may not be willing to give it up, or the others in the family may not be willing or ready to be free of domination. The most she can realistically hope for would be an improvement in the family's pattern of communication. Perhaps she can help them to talk *to* rather than *about* one another. (Thus, each time one family member talks about another in his presence, the nurse can turn to the other person for his reaction to what was said instead of replying to the first speaker in his own vein.) Perhaps she can assist them to use *words* to express their feelings and thoughts rather than violent *actions* (by asking the person who resorted to acting out his difficulties to relate what happened to him, and by asking him what he thinks might have occurred, had he talked about the incident instead of slamming the door, running away, or what not.) Hopefully, in the long run, improved verbal interchange will also lead to an improved balance of forces between the members of the family.

It is not easy to accomplish these results, however. First, many nurses feel a great sense of urgency to do something about the family member who is in need of nursing care and, therefore, will tend to pressure the key person in the family into trying to alter the situation rather than supporting him until he is ready to move on his own. Second, it is not always easy to recognize who wields the greatest power in the family. Family relationships are often very subtle and the person who seems to be the most powerful may turn out to be a decoy for the one who really "pulls the strings." Third, the nurse's own feelings about the various family members may cause her to take sides rather than remaining an impartial listener and facilitator for the entire group. The following illustrations may serve to elucidate these three points.

Effects of the nurse's pushing the patient into action

A young visiting nurse was assigned to visit a poverty-stricken family with seven children. The four youngest children all had birth defects, ranging from cataracts to clubfoot to a too-shallow hip socket to incomplete closure of the abdominal wall. The father worked sporadically, and drank on occasion. He stayed away from home as much as possible. Apparently, he could not bear the noise at home, or perhaps he could not tolerate the sight of his defective children. The mother was pregnant. The nurse planned to call on the family for the purpose of giving prenatal counseling to the mother and health supervision to the entire family. As she read through the available records, it became clear to her that she would have to move fast if she hoped to get the mother medical supervision in time to possibly save the unborn child from also being handicapped. She realized, too, that unless quick and effective help was provided for the children who had birth defects, they might not be able to enter kindergarten or have informal contacts with physically normal playmates, and that this might result in insuperable learning difficulties later on. She thought that as soon as these most important matters were taken care of, she would suggest that the mother take the three older children to the clinic for a health checkup and for immunizations which they might have failed to receive.

No wonder, then, that as soon as the nurse had obtained the necessary information concerning the mother's financial status, she immediately proceeded to impress upon her the importance of taking herself and the youngest children to the clinic at the first opportunity. It was not easy to converse with the mother, because six of the seven children were at home in the narrow, two-room apartment and their activities resulted in a considerable amount of noise. The mother had to interrupt the nurse frequently to admonish one or another of them, or separate two or three who were fighting for the possession of the same toy. Therefore, the nurse made sure before she left that the mother understood how important it was that she not delay her trip to the clinic. The mother said that she understood and that she would go the next day or the day after that.

The nurse felt a sense of relief when she left the apartment. Not only was she glad to escape the incredible hubbub, but she also felt that a step had been taken that might turn the tide in the health destiny of that family.

A few days later, the nurse returned to find out how the mother had fared at the clinic and, if necessary, to interpret anything that the clinic staff might not have made clear to her. It turned out, however, that the mother had not yet been to the clinic, because one of the children had a cold. She promised to go the following day.

The nurse returned at frequent intervals, always in the hope of hearing that the mother had taken herself and her youngsters to the clinic, but each time the mother presented another reason why she had been unable to go. Once she could not find a baby sitter for the older children. Once she had felt dizzy and thought she had better not venture out. The nurse asked the mother whether the husband could not help her out in this situation, but the woman ignored the suggestion and again promised that she would go soon.

The nurse simply could not understand the mother's quite obvious reluctance to get medical care for herself and her children. Why didn't her husband help her to get to the clinic, or at least insist that she go? Why did he avoid being at home when the nurse called, in spite of her frequent requests for a talk with him? Did these people have any idea of the seriousness of their problems? Finally, in desperation, the nurse asked the mother, "Doesn't it matter to you that you might bring another handicapped child into the world? Is this why you don't seem to want to seek all the help you can get that might possibly get at the root of your problems? Do you feel unable to go to the clinic alone? Would you like to have me go with you?"

The mother turned away from the nurse and said, almost inaudibly, that yes, it did matter to her whether the next baby would be handicapped or not and, no thank you, but she could and would go to the clinic on her own.

The nurse had lost confidence in the patient by this time so she talked the situation over with her supervisor. After hearing the story, the supervisor helped the nurse to understand that, certainly, after all these visits, the client could not possibly be uninformed, nor did she appear to be callous or feebleminded. Rather it seemed that she was under severe stress, what with seven little ones, most of whom had serious handicaps, the prospect of producing another, perhaps even more seriously handicapped child, and with no apparent support from her husband whose only way of coping with his tragedy was to get away from home. The supervisor pointed out to the nurse that pushing an apparently immobilized woman into seeking medical care, even though this would benefit both her and her children, could only add to her distress. She suggested that the nurse ask an older and more experienced colleague to accompany her on her next visit simply for the purpose of listening to what the mother had to say while the nurse would keep the children occupied so that the mother would not be distracted by them and could devote all her energies to the interview.

It did not take much urging to get the mother to talk about what was troubling her. She said that she had not wanted to become pregnant again, and that she had been terrified by dreams that the next child would be a two-headed monster. She dreaded her delivery and prayed to God to relieve her of her burden before it would come to term. She wondered what she could have done to cause her children to be born with handicaps and blamed herself for her present pregnancy.

Without even mentioning the need for the patient to visit the prenatal clinic, the older nurse asked the woman whether both nurses might come again in a few days so that they could talk further.

When they arrived for their third joint visit, the mother met them at the door and told them, with obvious relief, that she had been to the clinic, that appointments had been made for the handicapped children and that she herself had been examined. Although the physician had not promised her a healthy baby, he has assured her that, at the moment, everything seemed to be all right and that there was a good chance that the baby would not have any birth defects. He promised to follow her pregnancy closely, that he would do everything in his power to prevent complications, and that he would attend to her delivery himself.

This mother did not need the nurse to tell her what to do, or what would happen if she did not do it. In fact, the nurse's sense of urgency and the pressure she exerted on the mother to do something about her problem probably contributed to her inner turmoil and increased her inability to mobilize herself. What she did need was simply someone who would support her without judging her, in spite of her seeming inadequacy as a mother; someone in whom she could confide the terrible thoughts she harbored, her fears and her questions concerning her own guilt; someone who would not condemn her for these thoughts. As soon as she was given this kind of support, it did not take her long to assemble her forces and do what she knew she must do.

Finding the real family leader

How can the nurse be sure which of the family members is really the most powerful? At first, one person may appear to be the leader, then another, and finally a third. She can't always be sure, but she does have to start somewhere, so she lends her attention and interest to that person who appears to be the key figure at the moment; if the balance of power shifts in the direction of another member, the nurse will shift her main support to that person.

Several years ago, a public health nurse was assigned to visit a family that had come from eastern Europe. The 30-year-old daughter had recently returned home after having been hospitalized for two years with a diagnosis of chronic schizophrenic reaction, undifferentiated type. The aftercare clinic had arranged for this nurse's visits so she might help the family members with their readjustment to one another. It turned out that there was a considerable struggle for power going on between the daughter and the mother; the father seemed to be a helpless bystander. Specifically, the daughter stayed up all night watching television and then slept during the day. Whenever the daughter wakened, the mother cooked a separate meal for her, complaining bitterly all the while about how much extra work this meant for her. The daughter maintained that she was not well and that she was unable to sleep at night. Rather than getting herself upset by trying to go to sleep, she preferred to stay up until she became sleepy—usually about five o'clock in the morning. Then she would go to bed, sleep until about four in the afternoon, and then have breakfast. Naturally, she was not hungry at dinnertime. The father maintained that this was truly a tremendous burden for his wife, and that he was sure the daughter had not stayed up all night while she was at the hospital. When the nurse asked her about this, the daughter replied that at the hospital she talked with the attendants when she could not sleep; also, they gave her more medication than she was allowed to have at home. Besides, this was her home and she did not see why she could not do as she pleased.

When the nurse asked all three of them whether they had considered letting the daughter prepare her own meals, the mother became very agitated. She said that the least a mother could do for her sick child was to cook for her. All of the other children had left home and gotten married except this one—her baby. She felt that she needed to have some purpose in life, and cooking provided this. Only it was more than she could do to cook six meals instead of three. The husband smiled at the nurse and shrugged his shoulders. He indicated also that the daughter's upside-down schedule was a constant bone of contention between her and his wife, and that he was worried about the welfare of both of them. After all, his wife was no longer a young woman. On the other hand, he did not want to jeopardize his daughter's recovery because of strife over such a simple thing as meal hours.

As she listened to the pros and cons of their argument, it became clear to the nurse that the daughter was using the privileged status of her illness for the purpose of "getting even" with the mother, who had insisted upon babying her long after she had outgrown babyhood. In other words, the daughter was trying to assert herself against the irrational use of power by her mother, even though she was not doing it in a very constructive way.

It would have been unwise for the nurse to support the daughter's fight for autonomy openly. This would only have increased the mother's apprehension and resulted in greater effort on her part to keep her daughter dependent upon her. It was better procedure, therefore, for the nurse to become genuinely interested in the mother and try to find out what it was about the daughter's growing up that was so threatening to her. Hopefully, the nurse would then be able to alleviate the mother's fears to some degree so that she would not have to depend quite as much on her daughter for her own security.

During the nurse's next few interviews, the mother told the following story. She loved children and had always wanted to have a large family but, unfortunately, she had to have a hysterectomy early in her first marriage. At her husband's initiative, the marriage was annulled and, soon after, she met a widower who had four little children—her present husband. She promised him that she would be a good mother to the children and, indeed, she gave more of herself to them than she might have given to youngsters of her own. In fact, she did everything they asked of her and never disciplined them for fear of losing their affection of which she was not too sure anyway. The three older children, married now and with families of their own, had moved away from home as soon as they had found jobs. She said, with fortitude, that this was as it should be. The youngest one, thank goodness, preferred to stay at home, however, and let the mother take care of her. She had worked before "this thing" happened, but she did what she pleased with her earnings and payed her parents only a very small sum for her maintenance. The mother had encouraged her to go out on dates and to bring the young men home with her, so that she too could meet them, but the girl had always seemed to prefer to accompany her parents on visits to her brothers and sisters and to play there with her nephews and nieces. Then one day, out of the blue so it seemed, her daughter lost her job. Even though the reason for her dismissal had to do with company policies rather than with the quality of her work, she took it very much to heart. After that, she would not go out anymore, either for the purpose of finding another job, or for any other reason. She refused to accompany her parents when they went on vacation, and then, one day, she attempted to set the house on fire, and was placed in a mental hospital.

At this point in the interview, the mother became very tense; her face was flushed and she started to cry. The nurse encouraged her gently to go on with her story. Between sobs the mother said that her oldest daughter had blamed her for her sister's illness and had accused her of being the typical stepmother depicted in so many fairy tales. Crying bitterly now, she stressed again and again how much she had tried to be a real mother to the children.

After the mother had calmed down a bit, the nurse asked the patient, who had listened wordlessly to what had been said so far, whether she thought that her mother had acted like a stepmother toward her. The daughter shook her head and smiled. The nurse then asked the husband whether he thought she had. He protested that, on the contrary, he had to keep reminding her that she should think a little bit of herself and of him as well, and not only of the children.

The nurse then explained to her that even if she had been the young woman's real mother, the oldest daughter probably would still have accused her of being responsible for what had occurred, for most families find that it is very hard to accept emotional illness in one of their members. In their attempts to cope with what has happened, they look about for a reason—some event or some person on whom they may be able to pin the blame. It is not at all unusual for them to blame either themselves or another member of the family.

The nurse's words seemed to relieve the mother of a great burden. She dried her tears, took the nurse's hand and, practically forcing her to look into her eyes, asked her again and again, whether she had really meant what she had said, or whether she was just trying to comfort her. The nurse assured her that she had witnessed this phenomenon many times in her years of practice and that she certainly meant every word she had said. The mother sighed deeply several times and began to smile: "So it was really not my fault," she kept saying, as if to herself. "Of course it was not your fault," the nurse said, "nor anybody else's, for that matter." The mother looked up now and smiled at the nurse, the daughter, and the husband in turn saying, "It was not my fault; thank God it was not my fault." When the nurse left, the mother accompanied her to her car and once more squeezed her hand.

At the nurse's next visit she was told that the daughter, although she had in no way rearranged her sleeping pattern, was now preparing her own meals. It seemed that neither she nor her stepmother were any the worse for it; in fact, they both seemed to be considerably more relaxed. The nurse rejoiced inwardly, for it seemed that her course of action had proved to be right.

Her joy was short-lived, however, for gradually it became obvious to the nurse that, although mother and daughter engaged in frequent verbal arguments, they appeared to be relatively comfortable with each other. In fact, it almost seemed that they enjoyed these sparring sessions and appeared to be none the worse for them. At the same time, it also became apparent to the nurse that whenever the father spoke, the patient lowered her head, closed her eyes, and sometimes rubbed her forehead as if she were trying hard to return to reality. When the nurse encouraged her to reply or react to a statement her father had made she smiled apologetically and replied, vaguely, that she had been thinking about something else.

The nurse realized then, that the real power figure in the family, and the one who posed the most severe threat to the daughter's security, was the father who was operating behind the scenes, as it were. Therefore, the nurse attempted to focus her attention on him during their joint discussions. He said he wanted his daughter to get a job; that he and his wife were old people and would not be able to support her forever. When the nurse asked her what she thought about going to work again, the daughter said that she could not go out to look for a job because she did not have the right clothes to wear. Besides, she was not yet ready to work. She wanted to first get used to associating with people outside the family again. In the meantime, she would, before too long, start to take part in the group activities at the aftercare clinic.

The next time the nurse called, the father appeared to be extremely angry and was barely able to suppress his feelings. When asked what had happened, he retorted that his daughter had taken all her savings to buy herself new shoes, clothes and a winter coat, even though her closet was full of clothing she had bought before she stopped working and which was still practically new.

The nurse turned to the daughter who said, yes, she had bought herself new things because she wanted to look right when she went to the clinic and met all those new people. The nurse then tried to find out why the father thought it was so terrible that the daughter had bought herself a new outfit. Perhaps her old wardrobe was no longer in style? Besides, he had mentioned, had he not, that she had spent her own money?

At this point, the father's anger exploded with full force. She had enough clothes, he shouted. From now on, she was going to ask him first before she spent one penny, and if she ever squandered money on such foolishness again, he would see to it that she was readmitted to the hospital.

So that was it! Although the mother had certain needs which had, to some degree, hampered the daughter's growth toward independence, the daughter, however inappropriately, seemed to be able to hold her own with her. It was the father who, even though he appeared to be self-effacing and mild-mannered, represented the real threat to her. Hence, the daughter maneuvered to disassociate herself from the situation whenever he addressed himself to her because, by being passive and vague in her responses, she forestalled any argument with him. Apparently, her attempt to move toward health in her own way was extremely threatening to his power status.

When the nurse tried again to find out directly from him what it was about the daughter's purchases that enraged him so, he did not answer her. Instead, he got up, mumbled a few words about having an engagement and left the house. At her next few visits, he was absent and, when she asked the wife and daughter why he was not there, both seemed ill at ease and remarked that he could not stay home during the nurse's visits anymore because he had to attend to other, more important matters.

There was little doubt in the nurse's mind that the questions she had asked the father, or perhaps her manner of asking them, had threatened the father's power position with the family. To protect his position from future assaults by her he avoided presenting himself as a target. Apparently, he was confident that neither his wife nor his daughter would undermine his status in his absence, and he was right. The next few visits by the nurse yielded practically nothing. Although there was some discussion between the patient and her mother, apart from filling in time, it had little meaning for any of the participants.

When the nurse reported these new developments at the monthly aftercare team meeting, everyone agreed that there seemed little reason for the nurse to continue her visits at this time. Although her presence had been very helpful in the past, it now appeared to constitute a threat to the entire family, which, if kept up, might well lead to their losing the ground they had gained so far. It was decided that, instead, the social worker would ask both parents to come to his office so that they could jointly evaluate the daughter's progress since her return from the hospital, and formulate plans for the future. Having been forewarned about the father's feelings concerning his daughter's financial transactions, the social worker was prepared to proceed very cautiously, so as not to give him reason for another flight.

Could the nurse have known from the beginning which family member was really the most powerful? Probably not. She had to start her interaction with what presented itself to her, and it was only after she had dealt with what lay on the surface that the deeper and more dangerous aspects of the family power structure came to light. It was wise, therefore, for the nurse to first lend her support to the mother without actually taking sides in the struggle concerning sleeping schedules and meals. She was also correct in shifting the focus of her attention to the father when his powerful effect upon the daughter became clear to her.

I wonder, however, what happened when she tried to intervene between father and daughter. Was his need for leaving the field inevitable? I doubt it. I believe that, without her being completely aware of it herself, the nurse's emotions, instead of merely guiding her in her action, had gained the upper hand. And, instead of merely trying to find out what it was about the daughter's purchases that was so upsetting to the father, she obviously defended the daughter's right to use her own money as she saw fit. True, she did not express this openly, but the way she phrased her question may have left little doubt in the father's mind as to where she stood, and he sensed a conspiracy between the nurse and his daughter. He may have reasoned that since he could not permit an insurrection at this late date, and since he could not very well tell a nurse who had been sent by the hospital authorities to stay away, the only avenue open to him was to avoid seeing her.

This story illustrates what can happen when the nurse's own feelings cause her to take sides instead of listening impartially for the purpose of facilitating communication among members of the family. Of course, it is not only in the home setting that this sort of thing happens. It may occur in any group interaction in which the nurse happens to participate.

There is something about family interactions, however, that seems to make them more intense, more filled with emotion, than other interactions. Whether this emotion is expressed openly or carefully held in check, it seems to arouse, in turn, a disproportionate amount of affect in almost anyone who witnesses family interactions. One reason for this is that few people ever reach a stage of development that makes it possible for them to accept their family members as they are, without harboring unresolved resentments or unrequited wishes about the kind of people they would like their relatives to be. No wonder, then, that in her contacts with patients' families, the nurse may suddenly find herself being pulled into their struggle and, unwittingly, participating in it. This is especially true in situations in which the nurse comes from a background similar to that of the family, for she may have had to undergo a struggle for emancipation similar to that of the patient, and the person who holds the greatest power in the patient's family may remind her very much of the authority figure in her own.

Of course, it would be ideal if nurses were assigned to work with patients' families only after they had succeeded in resolving whatever conflicts they might have had with their own families but, for the present, this is a rather unrealistic expectation.

It is important, though, that every nurse who works with families have access to good clinical supervision in order to forestall deadlocks in the nurse-family relationship. It is also important that the nurse feel free to turn to her supervisor the moment she notices that her emotions toward one or another family member have assumed a personal hue or are out of proportion to the situation. As long as she is uncertain about what is happening within herself, the nurse will be wise not to press any issues within the family. This may seem to slow up her work for the moment but, in the long run, it will turn out to be the safer and faster approach.

Summary

We have seen, then, that the nurse-client relationship in the home is much more complex than it is in the more structured institutional setting. Even though she is called in on behalf of a patient, the nurse usually must deal with the family group as a unit. Besides having to be flexible as far as procedures and her own demeanor are concerned, she has to be alert to the shifting power structure among the family members and adapt her interactions accordingly. Further, her success in the home setting will require that she be aware of her unresolved feelings concerning members of her own family and her skill in keeping these feelings separate from what goes on in the work situation.

Although nurses usually practice in hospitals, long-term institutions or patient's homes, these are by no means the only work settings. A great deal could be said about the way working in a doctor's office, school, industry, or the armed services affects the nurse's relationships with her clients. However, going into detail about all these kinds of settings would carry us far beyond the scope of this book, the purpose of which is merely to indicate, and illustrate when necessary, the categories of factors that influence the nurse-patient relationship.

III

WHAT THE PATIENT BRINGS TO THE RELATIONSHIP

Chapter 10

Capacities for Experiencing What Is Happening

We stated earlier that the nurse-patient relationship focuses primarily on sustaining the patient in his experience (Chapter 6). We defined experience as a sequential process consisting of: 1) a person's perception of an inner or outer event or object; 2) his interpretation of this event in light of his perception, his past experiences and present state; and 3) his response to the interpreted perception, again in light of his past experiences and present capacities.

Let us now look at the implications that disturbances in these three subcategories of experience in the patient may have for the nurse's approach to him. These disturbances may be due to absence, incomplete development, or incapacitation of one or more of the components that constitute experience.

Absence of Capacity to Experience

An unconscious patient, for instance, is unable to perceive stimuli, to weigh or analyze them as to their meaning for him, and to respond to them in a way that would protect him from their influences. In other words, if deeply unconscious, he does not feel it if a foreign body penetrates his cornea. He cannot discriminate between hot and cold and therefore does not notice it if a hot water bottle, kept in his bed by a well-meaning member of the nursing staff following an operation, burns his skin. If his bronchial tubes are filled with mucus, he is unable to rid himself of this hazard by coughing it up.

Since the patient's capacity to experience is practically non-existent, it behooves the nurse to utilize her own capacities in his behalf. Thus, she must use her eyes, nose, skin receptors and ears in order to assess whether the patient's room is too brightly illuminated, too cold or drafty, too poorly ventilated or too noisy. She must decide on the temperature and speed of flow of his tube feedings. She cannot wait for him to tell her that his lips and tongue are parched, that he would like to turn on his side, that he has just wet his bed or that he is suffering from constipation. If ever there is an occasion when the frequently made statement, "The nurse must anticipate and meet the patient's needs," applies perfectly, it is when a patient is unconscious.

The unconscious patient is completely inert and, consequently, he behaves more like an inanimate object than a person. Therefore, the nurse must be particularly careful to keep in mind that he is a living human being. This is not always easy to do, especially if the state of unconsciousness persists for days or for weeks or months, as sometimes happens. In fact, the longer one's contact with a human being who seems unable to react in a human way, the greater the temptation to react to him as if he were the inert, heavy bundle which he appears to be.

One way of guarding oneself against giving in to this temptation is to keep in mind what the patient may have been like before he became unconscious and, hopefully, what he will be like again before too long. Another safeguard may be to think of what he represents to those close to him and what it means to them to know that he is being treated with all the respect to which they feel their loved one is entitled. In addition, the nurse can remind herself of what kind of treatment she would want given to one of her relatives who might be in a similar predicament. Finally, and possibly the most effective way of guarding oneself against treating the long-unconscious patient as if he were an inanimate object, is to talk to him as if he were capable of experiencing what is happening to him. Even though the nurse continues to anticipate his needs, she can address him by his surname, tell him what she is going to do and the reason for it, and check with him once in a while about what he might think of her measures. She cannot expect a response from him, of course, but, he may, at some level of his consciousness, take in the messages which she is trying to convey to him. It is possible that, even though he may not be able to form conscious images or ideas, his organism may register, in some way, that it has been handled with respect. As a result, if and when he does regain consciousness, his organism may not have to work through the effects of having been handled with disrespect in addition to the whole event of having been in this precarious state.

Perception

Absence of capacity to perceive

Let us now look at the patient who, although he is able to interpret and respond adequately, is lacking in one or another of his capacities to perceive. He may be blind or deaf. He may be lacking in heat or cold perception, or in kinesthetic sense. This lack may be congenital or it may be acquired. If it is congenital, its effect on the way that he interprets stimuli and responds to them is much greater than if his lack is acquired. Thus, the congenitally blind person creates for himself an image of a rose, say, that is likely to be quite different from that of a person who has lost his eyesight during middle age as a result of glaucoma. Similarly, no congenitally deaf person is likely to experience a symphony in the same way as Beethoven was able to do after he became deaf. Also, a person congenitally handicapped is usually better able to accept his condition, though he may be quite sensitive to people's attitude toward him. When a person loses one or another of his sensory capacities later in life, he has to cope not only with the loss of perception in this area, the newness of the state in which he finds himself and the adjustment which this entails for him, but he also has to learn to accept the fact that he may be perceived by others as belonging in a different category of people than he did in the past. This is likely to be especially difficult for him if he, himself, happens to have a prejudice against people belonging to this particular group. For instance, it is not at all unusual to hear an elderly lady who has lost her eyesight, and consequently has been put in a ward with similarly handicapped patients, explain to her visitors that the other patients are blind while she is merely unable to see. It is not unusual, either, that such a person will put up considerable resistance against participating in group activities with her wardmates or against attending braille-reading classes.

The nurse may expect, then, that the congenitally handicapped person is likely to respond to any widening of his perceptual field through alternate senses as if to a miraculous revelation. The person whose handicap is acquired, on the other hand, will probably first have to work through his loss before he can even begin to think of partially compensating for it through the use of his other senses. It would be unwise for the nurse to be particularly sympathetic to children who, from the outset, have not been able to see or hear, although she may be deeply affected by the realization of what these children are missing. It would be just as unwise for her to be so enthusiastic about rehabilitative exercises that she overwhelms the person who has recently lost his hearing, his eyesight, or his ability to sense where he is treading.

Whether the patient's condition is congenital or acquired, the nurse will need to provide the missing perceptions for the patient during the time when he has not yet learned to use other perceptive devices to substitute, at least partially, for his deficit. Thus, on entering a blind patient's room, especially if nurse and patient do not know each other well, she needs to announce herself by addressing him verbally. If she has never met the patient before, she may want to give him an opportunity to form an impression of what she looks like by letting him feel her face and also, perhaps, her hands, especially if she is to provide physical care for him.

Since the patient is likely to use his ears and skin as partial substitutes for his eyes, she must be particularly conscious of the ways that her steps, her voice, and her touch convey her emotional state to him. When a patient's senses are all intact, she can more easily attenuate a negative message, that she may have emitted inadvertently, through a positive counter message on another level. Thus, a nurse who is tired and eager to go home, may bump unintentionally against the patient's bed and cause him unnecessary discomfort. It may be easier for him to excuse her clumsiness if he can see her embarrassed, apologetic smile as well as hear her spoken apology.

While, in the beginning, the nurse should build in the missing perceptions for the handicapped person, she must not continue to anticipate the patient's needs indefinitely. Otherwise, he may not ever feel the necessity for learning to cope with his situation on his own. She does need to gauge carefully, however, how much frustration she will permit before intervening.

There may be days when the patient is likely to feel that he will never be able to remember where the different pieces of furniture are located, how to keep the socks which belong to each other paired, and how to find the right tie for the suit he is wearing. He may have forgotten how many steps there are to the bottom of the stairs and which direction to go to reach the front door. On such days, he may feel very sorry for himself, curse his fate and wish he had never been born.

The nurse must be careful that, while accepting his difficulties, she not display too much sympathy for him. Otherwise she would only encourage him to wallow in his misery and would thus increase the size of his already overwhelming load, rather than helping to lighten it. It might be better if she urged him to relax for a moment when he becomes discouraged and not to panic. The more upset he becomes, the less his chance for remembering what he does know. One way of helping him to regain his composure might be to offer him concrete help by handing him the right pair of socks, for instance, or tying his tie for him. Then, if necessary, the nurse can calmly review his training sessions with him another few times. She can remind him that he should not think of too many problems at once, that he should allow himself sufficient time for each task and think of the next one only after the previous one has been safely accomplished. She can also assure him that what he has learned is likely to come back to him when he needs it, especially if he trusts his capacity for recall rather than interfering with its process by doubting his abilities.

It will be easier for her to choose a suitable approach to her patient if she is aware of some of the characteristics that go along with certain perceptual deficiencies, or with the conditions that cause these deficiencies in the first place. It is well known, for instance, that people who are in the process of losing their hearing tend to be suspicious of what is being said around them, and that they tend to be more comfortable in one-to-one relationships than in groups where verbal communication comes at them from all directions and at unpredictable intervals.

I have often found that people who suffer from otosclerosis, tend to be high strung and tense, with a tendency to over-react to their rather unpleasant symptoms which, in turn, is apt to aggravate these symptoms. It seems to me, therefore, that the nurse can be particularly helpful to such patients if she approaches them in a calm, reassuring way, and if she can forestall any additional aggravation for them while they are waiting for the physician or for a hearing test.

It is well known to school nurses, for instance, that children who show little interest in their school work and who are inappropriately noisy and rambunctious, are frequently found to be suffering from a defect in vision or hearing. At first they try to make out what is written on the blackboard or what the teacher is trying to explain but, hard as they may strain their eyes or ears, they can catch only disconnected snatches of what is going on and, before long, they have been left behind their classmates. So they give up trying and, since just sitting there is rather boring, they start to amuse themselves in their own way. Instead of jumping to conclusions that a particular child who is not doing well in school has psychological difficulties (which, admittedly, he is likely to acquire if his present state remains unremedied), the nurse will do well to initiate eye or ear testing, or at least to check into the results of routine screenings.

Distorted perceptions

The nurse may also encounter patients who, instead of having an absence of, or a deficiency in, one or another area of perception, have a distortion in perception, resulting from a systemic condition or a deficiency in an organ itself. For example, anxiety and fatigue are likely to cause a narrowing of the perceptual field. A person learning to drive an automobile may find himself unable to look as far ahead as the speed of his car requires him to do. Similarly, one who drives on a turnpike for several hours at a stretch is likely to find himself focusing closer and closer to the hood of his car rather than hundreds of feet ahead of it.

When accidents happen, it is frequently found that the person involved has been unusually anxious or tired and simply did not see the danger as it approached, but became aware of it only after it had already made its impact. Nurses in all kinds of settings could do a great deal to prevent accidents if they provided opportunities for their co-workers and clients to discuss this phenomenon of narrowing perception during anxiety and fatigue, and if they could help them to respect it as a fact of life that must not be ignored (*see* Chapter 4).

It will be useful for the nurse to know that depressed patients tend not only to interpret the world as being dull grey, monotonous, and not worthwhile but that they actually perceive it as being so. For instance, their senses literally do not register the particular brightness of hues, which is so characteristic of clear fall days, and the clarity in which distant objects demarcate themselves—on such days—from their surroundings. The nurse may be less displeased with her patient's lack of interest in the beauty around him if she reminds herself that he is probably not even perceiving it.

It will also be useful to the nurse if she can remember that patients who suffer from schizophrenic reactions frequently perceive the world around them completely differently from the way those who are well perceive it. As a result of projecting the precarious state of their own personalities upon their surroundings, they may perceive the environment as if it might fall apart at any moment, or collapse upon them as the pillars of the temple did upon Samson. They are not very clear as to where their own boundaries end and those of the next person begin and it is not surprising, therefore, that sometimes they call themselves by another person's name. They also tend to perceive objects and thoughts in a fragmented way, as isolated patterns, without being able to put these fragments together to form an integrated whole—an experience which is, supposedly, similar to that which results from the ingestion of mescaline or LSD.

It is important, then, that the nurse does not discount the fact that the schizophrenic patient's perception is probably quite different from her own. His behavior and verbal communication, however bizarre in themselves, may well have meaning when they can be related to the ways in which he perceives his world. But, the nurse cannot expect the patient to make this meaning clear to her in terms of her own perceptions. Yet, this is what she is really trying to do when she cannot follow his trend of thought and asks him to "explain this" to her or to tell her "what this means." The patient finds that kind of instruction hard to understand and hard to follow, for after all the meaning of what he is communicating is perfectly clear to him (in light of *his* perception). It would be better if the nurse, when at a loss to know what he is trying to communicate to her, would ask him to tell her "what is going on now" or "what comes to (his) mind" in relation to what he has just said. This will probably bring her closer to his perception of what he is experiencing and, once she has that information, it will be easier for her to draw inferences as to what he is trying to convey to her.

Hallucinations

Patients with a toxic condition, or those with a very high degree of anxiety that is leading them in the direction of a psychotic break, or that has already resulted in a full-fledged psychosis, may tend to perceive their own thoughts and inner images as coming from the outside. The medical term for this phenomenon is hallucination. There are all kinds of hallucinations. Some are visual, some auditory; some are tactile, some olfactory. Some are terribly threatening and frightening to the patient; others are a pleasant pastime that he uses to occupy his idle time. There is certainly no single approach—on the nurse's part—that will apply to all situations in which patients hallucinate.

If the patient seems terrified by what he is experiencing in his misperception of his inner thoughts, the nurse should let him know that she and those working with her are not intimidated by whatever it is that is threatening him, and that they will see to it that he does not come to harm. She must be careful, however, not to inadvertently reify, i.e., not to make real, what is actually only a thought or an image. In other words, she must guard herself from saying to him that "we will not let *him* (or her) hurt you," or "all of us will protect you from your *voice*," for, unfortunately, it is usually a staff member who lends a body and thus greater reality to what had previously been perceived by the patient as merely an uncanny "shouting" or "pointing" or "whispering."

When the patient admittedly or covertly starts to hallucinate while he is with other people, it is usually a sign that he has had more interpersonal contact than he can tolerate at this time for, much as he may long to be with people, he is also deeply afraid of coming close to them. So, in order to protect himself from the people around him he turns to his inner radio, as it were. In such a case, it may be helpful for the nurse to give him an opportunity to get away from the group, or at least to try to deflect the group's attention from him for a while.

If he begins to hallucinate while he and the nurse are discussing matters of concern to him, it usually signifies that it is very uncomfortable for him to deal with this subject. It may help at this point if the nurse, rather than pursuing the topic further, will check with the patient as to his feelings regarding what is being discussed. If he admits to being uncomfortable, the nurse can check further into what it is about their talk that is making him so uncomfortable. She can also suggest that he not rush into discussing the topic, but rather that he take his time about it and stop for a while, if need be, whenever it seems to become too much for him. If he is not yet ready to admit that he is uncomfortable (he may not be aware of it himself or may not dare tell it to the nurse), the nurse might suggest to him that they defer further discussion until they meet again or that they take a short break so that he can get up and walk around a bit or go out for a drink of water. In time, he will probably use these ways of relieving his anxiety himself instead of having to resort to hallucinating in order to protect himself from it.

Patients who use their hallucinations as toys, so to speak, usually have been ill for a long time and have also been deprived of meaningful outer stimuli for years. Because of their lack of social skills, they tend to be very uncomfortable when with real people. And, since it is so much easier to control and predict the actions of benign hallucinatory figures than those of even the most benign flesh-and-blood person, these patients are likely to be quite reluctant to exchange their fantasy life for contact with living human beings. The nurse needs to understand this reluctance, and go very easy in her efforts to establish a relationship with this kind of patient. It will be best for her to spend only short periods of time with him, once or twice daily, and to keep herself distant enough from him physically so as not to overwhelm him with her presence. Also, it will be best for her to go along with the topic which he initiates or, if none is forthcoming, to suggest that he tell her about a pleasant experience he has had in the past or about something which he used to like to do. She can even talk about the weather, if these suggestions draw no response from him. If the nurse focuses the conversation too closely on him and his current life, or allows too long a period of silence, the chances are that he will become even more uncomfortable with her. In his deprived state, there is relatively little about his life that he may find worthy of relating to her. On the other hand, he is probably not ready to share his inner fantasy life with her. In dealing with this kind of situation, I have found that if a topic comes up that is amusing to both the patient and the nurse, it seems to break the ice and set the stage for the development of a meaningful relationship.

Unawareness of perceptions

One other phenomenon that I believe falls into the area of perception and which, to my knowledge, has received little attention in the nursing literature, has to do with a person's inability, or his neglect, to pick up clues (from his own organism) that would convey to him that he is not at ease. For instance, you may, at some time, have been engaged in a piece of work that for one reason or another, had to be completed that same day—mowing your lawn perhaps, or writing a report that was long over-due. You may have noticed that, although you may have had some twinges of discomfort, as long as you concentrated on what you were doing, you really were not aware of the fact that you had begun to feel very tired and that your every muscle was aching. It was only when you started to make mistakes, either by skipping areas of grass that should have been mowed or by skipping lines in transcribing your report into its final draft, that it occurred to you that something had been seriously amiss with you for quite a while. Or, have you ever been intently engaged in a conversation on a topic very close to your heart and noticed only after the other person had left that what he said had made you very angry?

This is not an unusual occurrence; it can happen to any of us whenever we feel that we must stretch our limits of endurance in order to meet an objective that is important to us. For some people, however, this phenomenon of not being aware of early warning messages sent out by their organisms, or of being only subliminally aware of them until after a precarious state of disequilibrium has been reached, is a way of life rather than the exception. These people are usually unaware of their lack of awareness. All they know is that they frequently suffer from the occurrence of certain sets of very undesirable symptoms or behaviors that seem to appear at the most inopportune times.

These symptoms vary in different people. Some may suffer from frequent, excruciating headaches. Others may periodically find themselves feeling very blue and will break into tears at the least provocation. Still others may experience states of almost intolerably painful fatigue, especially when in the presence of other people. There are also those who tend to erupt into violent fits of temper which are quite disproportionate to the events which preceded them.

The common element in these symptoms and behaviors is that they are most unwelcome and quite embarrassing to the person who exhibits them, yet he knows of no way to gain control over them. In fact, the more he tries to guard against their occurrence by trying to exercise his will-power, the more likely they are to display their autonomy.

Frequently, in order to avoid the unpleasant consequences that result from his uncontrollable behavior, the person will tend to restrict his life and avoid those occasions that are apt to bring on his symptoms. This may well lead to the appearance of his symptoms on occasions when they had not previously occurred, and to a consequent additional restriction of his life space. Since what is happening is so utterly unacceptable to the person, it may take him a long time to assemble sufficient courage to seek professional help. Some people may never get to the point of seeking help on their own, and are only brought to the attention of professionals after they have run into serious difficulties with themselves and others.

Most nurses have heard patients who were ready to be discharged promise that when they go home this time, they will turn over a new leaf. They will not yell at their husbands and children, even when they forget to wipe their shoes before they enter the hallway. Or they will do a little cleaning and ironing every day so that the housework will not accumulate to unmanageable proportions. Because the nurse knows the usual fate of most of these good intentions, she should not encourage this line of reasoning. Instead, before his discharge, she should try to help the patient to gradually develop a sense of awareness of what it is that happens to him before he must resort to his symptom.

Unfortunately, this is not an easy task. Not every patient is willing to look at his problem this way, nor does the philosophy of the setting in which he and the nurse find themselves always encourage this kind of self-appraisal. After all, it is more honorable and certainly less work for him to disclaim any responsibility for the idiosyncratic reactions of his organism, especially if he has definite ideas as to what he should and would be like if it were not for these reactions. Or, if he concludes that his behavior demonstrates that he is obviously no good, he may not see any purpose in trying to work at overcoming it.

If the patient is willing to make the effort to find out what is happening to him and if what he finds out is not in opposition to his therapeutic regimen, he and the nurse must be prepared for a series of frustrations and a number of recurrences of his symptom, for, much as he may strain to catch the messages his organism emits before the appearance of the full-blown symptom, he is likely to draw a blank at first. Should he have to be readmitted to the hospital because of a relapse of his symptomatology, both he and the nurse (not to mention his family and his employer) may, at first, feel disappointed. Hopefully, however, the nurse will soon realize that each apparent failure provides another opportunity to find further connections between the symptom and what has happened in his life, and be able to help the patient and his family to see this too.

Gradually, the patient will begin to notice certain recurrent patterns of events that precede the appearance of his symptom, and, even more gradually, he will begin to notice warning signs that tell him that not all is as it should be. First, he will pick up these signs only shortly before the symptom itself occurs, and probably too late to do something constructive about it. But eventually he will become attuned to his inner messages and will learn to become aware of them closer and closer to the time when they first make themselves known.

But this is not all the patient must learn to do. He must also learn to accept his organism's warning signs as legitimate limitations and to respect and heed them, regardless of whether he does or does not approve of them. Furthermore, he will need to develop skill in responding to his inner warnings and in standing by them in a way which, without being offensive, conveys his conviction to others as well as to himself.

As he develops and practices his skill in recognizing, accepting and standing by his limitations, he will find that, gradually, his symptoms occur less and less frequently. He will also find that the greater his ability to communicate his early reactions to himself and to others in a matter-of-fact way, without needing to be apologetic or defensive, the more others will tend to accept them without opposition or argument.

How the nurse can help the patient with faulty perceptions

Specifically, what is the nurse's role in these situations, apart from being patient and supportive? If the person is undergoing psychotherapy with another professional, the nurse needs to be careful that she does not, by her solicitude and willingness to listen, drain off information and energy from the therapeutic relationship. She can, however, suggest to the patient that a certain event which upset him during the day may well be worth reporting to his therapist.

If a patient who is not in psychotherapy with another professional, tells his nurse how, from now on, he plans to be a different person, she can indicate to him that she is skeptical as to the outcome of his intention, since willpower has little to do with the problem with which he is grappling.

If the patient continues to complain about his symptoms or his behavior, she might suggest to him that he think about the circumstances when they occur and that he discuss these with her at their next meeting. The chances are that he will first report the event that occurred and other people's part in it, as if he had not been present or as if he had, at most, been an innocent bystander. Gradually, the nurse can ask him about his participation in the event, and then about the thoughts that might have crossed his mind and what he might have felt at the time. Probably the patient will be unable to give her a full account of his actions, thoughts and feelings. This is to be expected, for otherwise he would not have found himself in his current predicament. The nurse can suggest, then, that on future, similar occasions, he not only concentrate on what others do but that he also begin to try to remember his own actions, thoughts, and concomitant emotions, and that they look at these together. (*See* Chapter 7).

Instead of feeling helpless and discouraged with himself, the patient will probably begin to develop an inquiring attitude with respect to his symptom as well as a certain amount of acceptance for his lack of skill. This attitude will be quite different from his previous one of self-condemnation or self-indulgence. Gradually, as he brings out more and more facts and begins to see connections between his unnoticed inner responses and his impulsive acts or incapacitating symptoms, he is likely to become enthusiastic about this kind of inquiry. As a result he may well develop a continuing interest in strengthening his sense of self-awareness and in assuming responsibility for the limits he must set for others and for himself. Of course, the fewer preconceptions the nurse has as to what people ought to be like, the better she will be able to guide her patients in developing skill in listening to, accepting and standing by that which they really are (*see* Chapter 1).

What kinds of problem areas that both nurse and patient may need to be prepared to face with reasonable equanimity are likely to turn up in such explorations? Usually, these areas have to do with discrepancies between what the patient would like to be and the realistic limitations which his organism interposes. More specifically, the problem areas usually have to do with the patient's ambition to endure or achieve much more than his organism is willing or capable of enduring or achieving; with the patient's unwillingness to recognize and express the fact that he is annoyed with what is, after all, not a socially acceptable emotion; and with his reluctance to stand by those personal idiosyncrasies of his that brand him as different from others and different from what he thinks others expect him to be.

It will take considerable patience on the nurse's part and, hopefully, concrete successes in the patient's life, to convince him of the fact that, in the long run, he will be less of a nuisance and burden to himself and others, if he will acknowledge and stand by the limitations that go along with his uniqueness than if he continues to succumb to incapacitating symptoms and embarrassing behaviors that result from trying to be what he is not.

Let us turn now from the area of perception to the second experiential component, *interpretation.*

Interpretation

The first phenomenon which comes to my mind is somewhat related to the one we have just discussed. Only, in this case, the person is aware of his inner distress, but unable to differentiate it clearly as to its nature. For instance, some people interpret whatever inner tension they may experience as hunger, or thirst or the need for a smoke. As a result, they will aim to appease the distress by the intake of food or alcoholic beverages, or by the smoking of a cigarette. However, since the source of their discomfort may be entirely unrelated to hunger, thirst or the craving for nicotine, their "remedial action" is not likely to be very effective but may, by adding to the original malaise, well be the beginning of a vicious cycle. We all know people who are viewed by themselves and their contemporaries as being compulsive eaters, drinkers or smokers.

The nurse works similarly with patients who are unable to

interpret their inner perceptions correctly as with patients who are not aware of their perceptions. That is, she guards herself from focusing too much on the patient's eating, drinking or smoking, much as she may feel the need to impress him with the noxious effects of his indulgence. Instead, she tries to help the patient to become more sensitive to the qualities of his inner experiences so that he may name them appropriately and then deal with them accordingly.

She hopes that, before too long, the patient will be able to realize that, although he receives messages from within that cause him to think of strawberry milk shakes, he is not really hungry at this time, but tired, and the milk shake does not represent so much food, but a "pick-me-up." Or, he may be really annoyed by his wife's ceaseless prattle and, rather than telling her to keep quiet and thus starting an argument, his mind conjures up an image of this smooth, substantial beverage which can soothe his crackling nerves. Or, it may be that what he really wants is to get out of his chair, stretch, and perhaps take a walk around the block to satisfy his need for a brief change of pace. A pleasant, cool, and rich drink is, at best, only a temporary substitute for motion. A milk shake will not bring him any closer to knowing the boss's reason for asking him to stop in and see him at eleven, even though it may assuage his inner flutterings for a while.

It is also to be hoped that the patient, once he knows what he really is experiencing, will learn to either endure or deal with his discomfort, according to its nature. Hopefully, for instance, he will learn that the only thing to do when he has to go to the bathroom is to go and get it over with, even though it may possibly disrupt the conversation at a social gathering; neither one more cigarette nor one more tidbit will substitute for this trip. He will, hopefully, also learn that although another highball may give him temporary relief from his anxiety, it does not alter the fact that his disobedient, teen-age daughter is still out, even though it is past 2:00 A.M.

I have used the word "hopefully" on purpose. It seems to me

that it is much easier to help a person become aware of his perceptions than it is to help him alter his stereotyped interpretations of them, or his responses to them. In the instances cited earlier in this chapter, we noted that the patient's symptom was deeply disturbing to him, but this is not the case here. It is true that he may loathe and fear the consequences of his indulgence, but while it lasts, it does give him a certain amount of pleasure and relief.

It is understandable, therefore, that at the slightest provocation, he will again resort to a habit which has given him at least temporary respite in the past. Of course he will probably be filled with self-loathing and will be disgusted with his lack of intestinal fortitude when he steps on the scale the next day, or finds that he is unable to think through a simple problem, or when his upper back muscles ache from the extra work they have to do in order to provide him with a minimum of oxygen. He will probably also resolve that, one of these days, he will make a clean break—perhaps even tomorrow morning. But, when tomorrow comes, just the thought of sticking to his resolution gives him a feeling of overwhelming uneasiness. He has difficulty in just getting through the day as it is, and he simply cannot afford to add to his problems deliberately by breaking his habit at this time.

We can see how important it is for the nurse not to be judgmental of the patient who, in many ways, is already his own most severe judge. Perhaps she can help him to develop some effective alternate ways of coping with his daily stresses or maybe she can at least help him to formulate goals for himself that are genuinely his own. It just might be that he realizes and really does not care that he is much too heavy, even though he knows that medical scientists warn against the complications that can arise from being overweight. Perhaps he knows, intuitively, that if it were not for his obesity, he might be ill with a much more serious condition. Perhaps he knows that if it were not for his occasional binges, no one could live with him. And perhaps he also knows that, unless he smokes two or more packs of cigarettes while at work, his anxiety level will be so high that he cannot concentrate at all and he might have to be fired. I do not know whether these are legitimate reasons, but is it the nurse's place to discredit them?

The nurse needs to know that although many of these kinds of patients are able to improve, they are especially prone to relapses. Whenever a new stress arises with which the patient has not yet learned to cope, or whenever his current stresses seem to become less manageable (as, for instance, during the ten days preceding a woman's menstrual period), the patient is apt to interpret this experience in his favorite manner and to alleviate it accordingly.

The nurse can be of great help to the patient if she can show him that he need not be discouraged about his relapse and that he might, in fact, even have reason to be grateful that it has occurred, for it may well be his way of indicating to himself that something is going on inside of him which requires his urgent attention. It is important, therefore, that instead of continuing in his vicious cycle and having to suffer all the inherent consequences, he plan to get off his treadmill as soon as he can for just as long as it might take him to take stock of himself. Once he has listened to himself and regained his inner balance, he may find that he is operating on a higher level than he had been before the recurrence of his habit.

Lack of ability to accept experience

Sometimes a person can perceive and interpret his experience correctly for what it is, but he conceives of it as utterly unbearable. Therefore, his primary concern is not to deal with the experience in some way, but to rid himself of it at all costs, even if this means getting rid of the object which is generating the experience or of the subject which has to suffer it. It is hard for an outsider to assess whether the experience is really so terribly overwhelming for the other person. What matters is that the person involved interprets it as such and that, unfortunately, he often responds accordingly.

Nurses react to this phenomenon in their clients in a variety of ways. They may be just as deeply shocked at a crime committed by a parent who could not stand the helplessness generated in him by the constant crying of his 3-year-old child, as anyone else would be. At other times they may find themselves inwardly agreeing with an incurable or chronically depressed patient that perhaps he would be better off if he were dead. There may be other times when nurses become quite impatient with a client who claims that he cannot tolerate one more minute of what seems to them to be a minor complaint.

When the nurse finds herself reacting in any one of these ways, she must be careful not to let her emotions becloud her judgment. In order to prevent this from happening, it might help her to remember that she has a job to do—a job that involves helping the patient, if at all possible, to increase his tolerance for discomfort, which, by the way, has nothing to do with gritting one's teeth and "trying to bear it." On the contrary, stiffening up in order to brace oneself against discomfort does just the opposite of what it is supposed to do: It contracts one's capacity for tolerance, or at least sets a rigid boundary for it, instead of making it elastic or enlarging it.

Since the pain is there and clamoring to be acknowledged, it would be better for the patient if he could open himself up to his experience, to even let himself be inundated by it without, however, allowing it to wash him away. This is a tall order and whether or not it can be carried out will depend partly on the relationship between the magnitude of the experience and the patient's capacity for endurance. The latter depends, in turn, upon his past training as well as his basic attitudes. If his attitude is such that he believes what he is undergoing is not fair to him, or if he believes that he is entitled to be exempt from having to suffer and nobody and nothing has the right to force him to suffer, it won't be easy to try to help him and attempts to do so probably will not succeed. Perhaps the nurse can explain to him, during times when he is not suffering, that everybody seems to have his share of pain, and that apparently he is no exception. Maybe he can hear, understand and accept her explanation. Or, a religious advisor may be able to help. Later, when he is suffering severe discomfort, perhaps the nurse can remind him of what had been said and can stand by him as he begins to try to accept what is happening to him.

Sustaining a patient in his suffering

If he steadfastly refuses to accept his own suffering, however, the nurse must be extremely careful that no one, including the patient, comes to harm at those times when his experience is more than he is able or willing to tolerate.

Some concrete ways of helping a patient to tolerate his experience is to ask him to take a deep breath; to think of each instant as it comes instead of making long-range plans which are, naturally, colored by the blackness of the moment; and to take on what is coming at him instead of stemming himself against it with full force.

Some people, instead of living through their experiences, attempt to control them by trying to figure out why they are happening to them. As a result, the emotional impact of an experience continues to hang on, like an unfinished symphony. The nurse should try to encourage such a patient to consciously try to stop himself from thinking about the cause of his pain. Instead, if at all possible, he should try to concentrate on what he is experiencing and to participate in it. True, this will temporarily increase his pain, but it will also help it to subside. Afterwards, when he has come out at the other end of his suffering, so to speak, will be the time to take stock of what has happened and to learn from it.

I am sure that all nurses are familiar with what I am talking about and have themselves sustained patients through experiences which, perhaps, they thought the patients would not be able to endure: for some nurses it may have been assisting a patient to swallow a Levine tube or to undergo a lumbar puncture; for others it may have been standing by a patient who was being weaned from heroin without palliative medication. Some nurses may have had occasion to be involved in trying to comfort parents whose only child had just died from leukemia. Others may have worked with patients who, the moment they felt the least bit anxious or bewildered, were liable to assault their fellow patients or the ward personnel. And I am sure there are few nurses who have not been in the position of having had to wrestle by word or action with patients who felt they must rid themselves of the life which had become unbearable to them.

Effects of inability to interpret stimuli

Some patients, although able to perceive stimuli and to respond to them, may have difficulty in making sense of what these stimuli are all about. This may be due to the fact that they are unfamiliar with the stimulus or it may be due to a clouding of consciousness. Most nurses have seen senile patients who, dimly aware of the tension in their urinary or anal sphincter, but not quite clear as to what this tension signifies, vaguely fumble with door knobs in the hope, perhaps, of finding a bathroom, or at least some kind of release. Most nurses have also had experiences with postoperative patients who attempted to climb over the siderails of their beds, and with patients with delirium tremens who have tried to leave the premises via a window on the seventh floor. When these patients are asked where they are going, they will probably look blankly at the questioner and murmur something to the effect of "where else but out?" If the nurse explains to them that they are not allowed "out" and leads them back to where they came from, the chances are that the moment she turns her back, they will be on their way again.

Since these patients have difficulty in interpreting what is going on, they are sometimes deeply frightened and bewildered, and it is important that the nurse have some idea as to how she can reduce both their discomfort and the danger to which they may unwittingly expose themselves. It will help if she has some inkling of what the patient is perceiving that causes him to be so distressed. Does he have pain? Does he need a urinal? Or is he longing for a glass of ice-cold water? Is it that he simply has no idea where he is and how he came here in the first place? Is he, perhaps, terrified by ominous, moving shadows in his room or by whisperings coming from the corridor?

By trying to feel herself into the patient and getting some idea as to the source of his discomfort, the nurse can be of immeasurable help to him. It is amazing how favorably patients tend to respond to a proffered cool drink or a urinal placed in the right position. Usually, as soon as the cause of their tension is removed, they settle down peacefully and may even go to sleep.

By keeping the room light enough that the patient can clearly differentiate the objects in it, and by insisting that people in his vicinity either speak loudly enough so he can understand them or not at all, the nurse can considerably reduce the patient's opportunity for misinterpreting what he sees and hears. These measures, too, will usually help the patient to relax and even to drop off into much-needed slumber.

The situation is not quite as simple if the patient is restless and rambunctious because he does not know where he is, or whether it is yesterday or tomorrow. To be disoriented is very frightening to a person and he may, therefore, want to find his bearings at all costs. If he appears bewildered, the nurse should tell him where he is and why, and also what time of day or night it is. She can even assure him that within a few hours, he will be able to talk with the doctor, and with his family, and (if it is true) that he will probably be allowed to go home within days.

Usually, the patient responds to the nurse's explanations with gratitude and relief and abandons his effort to get away. The nurse needs to know and anticipate, however, that this peaceful state is not likely to last very long for, due to his brain damage, his overwhelming anxiety or both of these factors, the patient will probably not remember what he is told. It should not be surprising to the nurse, therefore, that moments after she has finished explaining his whereabouts to him, the patient again acts as if he had never heard of them. If the nurse understands the patient's inability to retain information, she will not be unduly frustrated over the fact that she has to repeat the same explanation again and again.

Let us move on now to the third and last component of experience as we have defined it, i.e., the patient's capacity to *respond.*

Response

Lack of capacity to respond

Every nurse has probably, at one time or another, had occasion to take care of a patient who, for physical or emotional reasons was unable to move and, consequently, was unable to communicate his needs either through verbal or nonverbal channels. Undoubtedly, in such a case the nurse, herself, experiences some of the patient's sense of frustration and helplessness. Knowing that the patient, in spite of his inability to communicate, is fully aware of what is going on and is able to interpret it appropriately, the nurse may not feel free to use her own judgment and simply go ahead with his care as if he were unconscious. However, if he is to participate in his care, the nurse must have some idea of what his needs are, and whether what she is trying to do for him is worth while.

Since both the sending out of a message and the acknowledgment of its receipt are necessary for successful and satisfying communication, and since the patient who is seriously handicapped in his ability to respond is lacking in both these areas, we can see why he as well as his nurse may succumb to feelings of frustration and helplessness.

What can the nurse do, then, to overcome this barrier? First, I believe, she must guard herself from appearing as all-knowing or even "knowing better" than the rest of the nursing staff on the ward. It may well be that another staff member who happens to be on a lower echelon of the nursing hierarchy has found some way of communicating with this patient. The nurse should, by all means, try to elicit the help of this person and not consider it beneath her dignity to learn from him.

If there is no one about who knows the patient well, the nurse may have to come to some agreement with him as to how they will communicate, before she even starts to give him care. She will try to find out from him whether there is some way in which he can convey "Yes" and "No" responses to her, perhaps by closing one eyelid, perhaps by moving his eye up, down or to one side, perhaps by the slightest twitch of a finger or toe or of one corner of his mouth.

Together with the patient, she will establish that this minute, hardly perceptible motion on his part will indicate that he means "yes," or "no." The nurse must, of course, formulate her questions carefully. She cannot simply ask him, "What would you like for dinner today?", for he has no way of responding to the question as she phrased it. She can, however, inform him that there are three choices on the menu: broiled fish, fried fish and boiled fish. And she can tell him that she will call off each item separately and will expect a "Yes" or "No" sign from him for each item.

Sometimes the patient may, by a faint, but unintelligible sound, indicate to the nurse that he is in distress. In order not to prolong his agony unduly by listing all possible reasons which might be causing his discomfort, the nurse needs to make some educated guesses right from the start. It is possible that the patient is lonely and even that he would very much like to discuss with the nurse the impact of his paralysis on his marital life. But probably these were not the needs for which he had tried to attract her attention. The chances are much greater that he had signaled her so she would help him to get back into good body alignment, or rid him of the fly which keeps settling down on his forehead. It may be that his nose is itching or that he wants her to wipe the perspiration from his face and neck. The nurse can tell the patient what she has observed and, by listing her observations, one by one, elicit from him through the faint "Yes" and "No" gestures of which he is capable, which one of these has priority.

If it turns out that she has guessed wrong and something else seems to be bothering the patient, the nurse must watch herself so that she does not become flustered, for the more tense she becomes, the less the likelihood that she will be able to pick up the clues that present themselves, and vice versa. The more at ease she can be with the patient, and the less concerned she is with her fear that she may not understand him and with her need to show him that she *can* understand, the greater the possibility that she will soon become just as attuned to his needs as some mothers are to those of their preverbal child.

With the patient who lacks the ability to respond, just as with the patient who is deaf or blind, the nurse must not let his handicap spill over into the way in which she appraises his other faculties. In other words, even though the patient is blind, or mute or paralyzed, he is still able to hear what she says; therefore, there is no need for the nurse to raise her voice. He is also perfectly able to think as an adult; hence, there is no need to address him as if he were of kindergarten age. In addition, the nurse needs to be careful that her solicitousness toward the paralyzed patient does not thwart, or even stifle, his striving toward some degree of autonomy.

Exaggeration of responses

Sometimes the problem is not so much one of *absence* of response on the part of the patient but one of exaggeration. An exaggerated response often manifests itself by destructive motor activity, which ends up with someone getting hurt and with some form of punishment for the patient. This happens frequently with retarded children and with those patients who need to deal with their discomforts on a motor reflex level without letting them have access to their frontal lobes.

Usually, these patients' destructive action can be controlled to some extent by a tranquilizing medication and by the holding out of reward and punishment, although neither measure solves the more basic problems which underlie these actions. Yet, with at least two of these underlying difficulties, the nurse can be of immeasurable help to her clients: One has to do with the patient's inability to use words and the other with his unawareness of the fact that one can release energy just as well by "building" as by "tearing down."

I once had the opportunity to observe how, within two weeks, nurses were able to help a group of institutionalized retarded children to abandon their frenzied activity, at least during the time they were together. At first, while the nurses merely observed them, these little 8-to-11-year-old boys dismantled within minutes every single object in the room that would come apart. Then the nurses introduced mechanical toys which the children could not only take apart but also reassemble. The way their overactivity and their destructive actions decreased in proportion to their increase in ability to put the parts together, was dramatic. The nurses also taught these children the words which denoted the emotional expression they were manifesting—such words as "I am hungry," "I am angry," "I want to play." Before long, instead of literally pulling each others' hair out and hitting one another over the head with whatever objects they happened to be holding, these little boys began calling each other names and telling one another how they felt about their toys being snitched away from them. And, of course, they were utterly delighted with their new skill.

I also had the opportunity, in that same institution, to observe how nurses were able to help a group of adolescent and late-adolescent retarded girls to cut down on their excessively seductive behavior by teaching them to use words instead. These girls had been used to expressing their liking for the staff, also their exasperation with them, I presume, through physical overtures which were utterly repulsive to their caretakers. In response, the staff would either lecture them, shoo them away, or punish them. The positive effect of these measures on the patients was minimal, however; they may even have proved enticing for some.

Then the nurses changed their tactics and, during special group sessions with these girls, taught them to say what they felt through the use of words rather than through bodily actions. If they felt they had to get physically close to a staff member, they were allowed to hold his or her hand, but kissing and embracing were out. They could tell the staff member that they liked him or her as often as they liked. They were even permitted to tell the staff that they would love to get close to them physically, and how close. But "acting out" was definitely forbidden. And, lo and behold, within days, the youngsters settled down and began talking about matters that genuinely concerned them, such as their fear of electric shock or their feelings about being called "low grades," and they even raised questions about what would become of them in the future.

Nurses can extend the same kind of help to non-retarded clients who tend to use their arm and leg muscles toward each other or the staff, instead of their vocal cords. Usually the results will not be quite as dramatic as in the two instances described above, but they can certainly be gratifying both to the patient and the nurse.

In this chapter I have tried to give some examples of ways in which patients can be handicapped in their capacities for experiencing what is happening to them, and to point out certain principles of approach for the nurse which apply to certain categories of these handicaps. In the next chapters I should like to consider selected factors which may have bearing upon the way in which the patient can and wants to use the capacities which are available to him.

Suggested Readings

Boss, Medard. *Psychoanalysis and Daseinsanalysis.* New York: Basic Books, 1963.

Bruch, Hilde. *The Importance of Overweight.* New York: W. W. Norton & Co., 1957.

Burd, Shirley F., and Marshall, Margaret A. (eds.). *Some Clinical Approaches to Psychiatric Nursing*. New York: The Macmillan Co., 1963.

Huxley, Aldous. *Doors of Perception and Heaven and Hell*. New York: Harper & Bros., 1954.

Jung, Carl G. "Psychogenesis of Mental Disease" in *Collected Works, III. New York;* Pantheon Books, 1953.

Kasanin, J. S. (ed.). *Language and Thought in Schizophrenia*. New York: W. W. Norton & Co., 1964.

Keller, Helen. *The Story of My Life*. New York: Doubleday & Co., 1954.

Morgan, J. "Care of Hallucinated Patients," *Nursing Times 60* (Oct., 1964), pp. 1323-1324.

Ruesch, Juergen. *Disturbed Communication*. New York: W. W. Norton & Co., 1957.

Schwartz, Morris S., and Shockley, Emmy Lanning. *The Nurse and the Mental Patient*. New York: John Wiley & Sons, 1955.

Searles, Harold F. *Collected Papers on Schizophrenia and Related Subjects*. New York: International Universities Press, 1965.

Sechehaye, M. A. *Autobiography of a Schizophrenic Girl*. New York: Grune and Stratton, 1951.

Straus, Edwin W. *Phenomenological Psychology*. The selected papers of Erwin W. Straus, translated, in part by Erling Eng. New York: Basic Books, 1966.

Ujhely, Gertrud B. *The Nurse and Her Problem Patients*. New York: Springer Publishing Co., 1963.

Ujhely, Gertrud B. "Basic Considerations for Nurse-Patient Interaction in the Prevention and Treatment of Emotional Disorders," *Nursing Clinics of North America I*:2 (June, 1966), pp. 179-186.

Watts, Alan W. *The Wisdom of Insecurity*. New York: Pantheon Books, 1949.

Watts, Alan W. *This Is It and Other Essays on Zen and Spiritual Experiences*. New York: Pantheon Books, 1960.

Chapter 11

The Patient's Condition and the Meaning it Has for Him

Two of the most crucial factors that influence the way a person is likely to perceive, interpret, and respond to what is happening to him are his *condition* and what his condition *means* to him. His condition represents the particular state of physiological, psychological and—nowadays—sociological disequilibrium in which he finds himself. This state manifests itself in a cluster of signs and symptoms which follow a lawful course from their etiology to their eventual outcome, and is defined by such diagnostic terms as pemphigus, schizophrenic reaction or myocardial infarction.

Although the last chapter dealt primarily with disturbances in the capacity to perceive, interpret, and respond, the patient's condition was frequently referred to as being intimately related to these disturbances. For example, glaucoma and otosclerosis were mentioned as causing loss of visual and auditory perception, and depression and schizophrenia as being the basis for distortion in both perception and interpretation of the world. Difficulties in response were seen as stemming from damage to the nervous system caused by such conditions as delirium tremens, cerebral arteriosclerosis and trauma. There are innumerable additional examples of conditions that affect the patient's capacity for experience—the olfactory hallucinations caused by certain brain tumors, the paranoid ideation which usually accompanies the metabolic disease porphyria, and the frantic overactivity frequently associated with one kind of thyroid disease.

Factors Influencing the Meaning the Patient's Condition Has for Him

The meaning his condition has for a person depends upon a multitude of factors which include his past experience with the condition and his current knowledge about it. They include also his expectations from life which, in turn, depend partly upon his age, his cultural background and social status (*see* Chapter 1). They include further (and here we come full circle to where we started) the patient's capacity to perceive, interpret, and respond to what is happening to him and the condition itself.

Let me explain this by an example. Suppose a person is suffering a myocardial infarction. If his father had died young from the same condition, the patient, apart from being seriously ill by virtue of the condition itself, may "know" that this means the end for him, even though the location and extent of the myocardial damage does not justify his dire prediction. However, because of his conviction, based on past experience, the patient may perceive any minor discomfort as being more severe than its objective manifestations would lead others to believe it to be. And so, regardless of the medical evidence, to the patient his discomfort is a sign that he will soon die. Consequently, he is likely to respond to his discomfort with either increased alarm or complete resignation.

If a 35-year-old patient has never been told that myocardial infarctions can and do happen to men of his age, he may interpret his severe precordial distress as a stomachache resulting from his having eaten too much for dinner. Therefore, he may not seek medical assistance while there is still time for him to benefit from help.

A person who sees himself as someone who is never ill (and, perhaps, must not be ill), may also tend to ignore, as long as he can, the premonitory signs and symptoms which frequently precede a myocardial infarction, until he collapses—wherever he may be. If found in time and given immediate care, he will probably ridicule any medical warnings and not cooperate with the regimen of rest the physician may try to impose on him.

Again, a lonely, 80-year-old widower in a nursing home who suffers a heart attack is probably less threatened by it than a 40-year-old father of young children who has just been promoted to the vice-presidency of his firm. His usual personally and culturally prescribed pattern of perceiving, interpreting and responding to discomfort will help to determine whether he seeks medical attention or not, whether he will exaggerate or minimize whatever discomfort he feels, and whether he will be alarmed by it or take it in his stride. And yet, while the person is battling for his life, the vitality of his organism, or the lack of it, and the seriousness of the attack itself may possibly override all these other considerations. Thus, while he is suffering agonies of pain and fighting for every breath, any meaning of what is happening to him may be suspended for the time being except that of "survival" for some, and, for others, "death."

There seems, then, to be a reciprocal relationship between the patient's condition (and its meaning to him), and his capacity to experience. Or, to phrase it somewhat differently, while his condition and its meaning to him may very much affect the patient's capacity to perceive, interpret, and respond, his perception and interpretation of his condition and his response to it may, in turn, well determine its outcome.

Although in itself a truism, this statement, as formulated here, has, I believe, tremendous implications for nurses. As members of one of the healing professions, nurses share in the over-all obligation to do everything in their power to foster a positive outcome of the patient's *state*; and as members of the nursing profession, they have the specific responsibility, I think, of sustaining the person in his *experience* (*see* Chapter 6). Therefore, whether they are aware of it or not, nurses have a potentially crucial role to play with respect to both axes of the patient's predicament—his experience and his condition. By lending knowledgeable physical and emotional support to the patient, and by skillfully carrying out delegated medical tasks and nursing procedures, nurses can exert a favorable influence upon the way in which the patient perceives, interprets, and responds to his condition as well as upon the condition itself; and since these two factors influence each other, her positive influence upon one of them may well lead to improvement in the other.

Furthermore, by trying to gain an idea of what his condition means to the patient and, if possible, helping him to correct any misconceptions he may have concerning it, the nurse may be able to disrupt much of the negative interaction that may occur between his state and his experience of it.

There is no doubt in my mind that the nurse can make a most valuable contribution, not only to patient care but also to knowledge about patient care. This contribution is partially based upon knowledge from medicine and the biological and social sciences and its application. It is also based upon autobiographical and fictional accounts in the literature and, last but not least, upon the nurse's own observations and personal experience with similar conditions in others and, possibly, herself. In addition, since the nurse, by virtue of her professional role, can have an impact both on the patient's condition and his experience of it, it is up to her, I believe, to be knowledgeable not only about interrelationships between the two, but also, about ways of influencing these interrelationships in a positive direction rather than a negative one.

Interrelationship between the Condition and the Patients' Experience of It

Of course, there are innumerable ways in which the patient's condition (and its meaning to him) and his experience can interact with one another. And there are also many ways in which one can look at these interactions in an attempt to find common denominators from which some principles of approach for the nurse might be derived. The following is a description of one such attempt.

Let us consider the interrelationship between the patient's

condition and his experience as falling into one of five broad categories: One, the patient is overwhelmed by his condition; two, he protects himself from conscious awareness of it by irrational mechanisms of escape; three, although aware of his state, he is unable or unwilling to accept it; four, he uses his condition for ulterior purposes; and five, he accepts his condition.

Before going further into this classification, we should note that sometimes examples of all five categories may occur in one and the same patient, in orderly or unordered sequence. Sometimes, most of the patients suffering from a specific disease experience it in one typical way. Other patients experience whatever happens to them in a manner which is characteristic for them (or people of similar background) but which is not necessarily characteristic for their condition.

Now let us take a brief look at each of these categories and see what principles for nursing we can derive from them.

He is overwhelmed by his condition

When the patient's condition (or its meaning to him) is so overwhelming to him that his whole being is flooded by it, he finds it impossible to defend himself against its impact. This may be due to the nature of the condition itself as, for instance, in cases of stroke, typhoid fever, or a severe state of depression. It may be due not so much to his condition's current effect upon the patient but to what he anticipates its effects to be in the perhaps not too distant future as, for instance, when he is told (or finds out, somehow), that he has multiple sclerosis, schizophrenia, or an incurable kidney disease. Or, the patient may be overwhelmed not so much because of the intrinsic harmfulness of his condition but because of its implications for his view of himself. Thus, a man who is rejected from the military service of his choice because of a slight curvature of his spine, or because he is unable to see objects stereoscopically, due to a defect in the coordination of his eye muscles, may feel utterly defeated; he sees the rejection as proof that he lacks virility.

Similarly, a woman who, close to her menopause, must have her uterus removed because of fibroid tumors which cause her to bleed excessively, may be completely shattered by having to acknowledge the fact that from now on she will not be able to bear a child.

How can a nurse help the patient who is overwhelmed by his state? It seems to me that, regardless of the source of the patient's reaction, the nurse needs to care for him as she would for any patient who is utterly *helpless*. That is, initially, she must anticipate, or at least recognize, his needs and meet those which are within her power to meet without waiting for the patient's call. This will convey to him that, although he is helpless and unable to summon help, he is not without a reliable source of strength from the outside and therefore is not abandoned. As a result, the patient may not have to seek refuge from his helplessness by resorting to thoughts of utter despair and hopelessness. The more gentle but competent the nurse is in the way she handles equipment as well as the patient's body, the greater the chance that he can give in to his helplessness without becoming panicky about it and the more likely that, as a result, he will be able to rally his resources and eventually manage to remobilize himself.

It happens quite often, however, that, even though the patient feels better after a while, and his condition improves to some extent, he continues to cower in a corner as it were, unable to come out of his immobilization. In addition, he is frequently quite resistant to any attempt by the nursing staff to get him to move about. It is as if he has become marooned in his inertia and as if the world around him, seen from his current perspective, is assuming increasingly gigantic proportions that he feels less and less able to cope with.

In such a case, the nurse cannot simply sit back and wait for the patient to take the first step, for the chances that he will assume the initiative in the near future are likely to decrease, while the chances of dangerous sequelae such as pneumonia and muscular contractures, or even permanent loss of contact with his former environment, increase with every day that passes. It is imperative, therefore, that the nurse help the patient to mobilize himself even if this should be against his will. She may have to insist that, with her help, he get up and that he walk with her along the corridor or outside on the grounds, even if only for a few minutes. She may have to insist, further, that he attend prescribed activities although he should not be forced to take an active part in them. If he cannot walk, he should, if at all possible, be wheeled out in a chair or even on a stretcher, and his attention should be drawn to objects outside himself such as a sunset or a cloud formation, a tree in bloom, the antics of a squirrel, or a tugboat passing by on the river.

If his fear of leaving the security of his bed is so great that his resistance to being moved from it is insurmountable—barring a physical struggle—the nurse should at least move his limbs passively to a full range of motion and should introduce him to new stimuli that can be brought into his narrow range of interest. For instance, she can move his bed to another place in the room, and thus expose him to a different view of his surroundings. She can also turn on a radio or television set for short periods of time, or look through a magazine with him while at the same time making comments about the pictures.

It is understood, of course, that the nurse will keep in mind the real difficulty that her well-meaning attempts to help him may present for the patient. She must guard herself, therefore, from being too enthusiastic. On the other hand, if she is to help him to overcome his resistance, she cannot afford to act too sympathetic with his plight. It will sustain her to remember that, if she perseveres in her efforts, the patient will sooner or later reap worthwhile rewards. Gradually, he will begin to break down the walls of his prison in which his inertia keeps him confined and, as a consequence, the world that had loomed as a dangerous giant around him will slowly resume a more manageable size. It is to be hoped, in addition, that the day will come when the patient will no longer be the victim of his condition and completely at its mercy, but will ally himself to those inner and outer forces that have tried to liberate him from its hold.

Unconscious patient. A specific example of a condition that would fall into this category is found in the patient we discussed in Chapter 10—the one whose total organism is taken over by his condition to such an extent that he is unable to defend himself against noxious stimuli and unable to make his wants known, except indirectly through such signs as bedsores, elevated blood pressure, or mucus in his throat. We noted that this may occur when the patient is unconscious, and may be due to a variety of reasons. We also stated that the nursing principle to be applied here is anticipation of the patient's needs while resisting the temptation to treat him like an inanimate object.

The immobilized patient. Sometimes, the patient may be able to perceive and interpret what is happening to him but not be able to respond to it. This happens in patients who have had a cerebrovascular accident, or who have certain disorders of the nervous system; it can also happen in those patients with schizophrenic reactions who are paralyzed by a catatonic state. The patients in this second group are not quite as helpless as those in the first—at least not after the initial impact of their state—because they can register (and usually quite accurately) what goes on around and within them, even though they cannot respond to these happenings.

The nurse needs to keep in mind the terror experienced by a person whose mind may be quite clear, a person who has been able to take care of his own affairs and perhaps the affairs of others also, but who suddenly finds himself completely helpless to the extent that he cannot formulate or express his needs. She must also be aware of the mounting frustration in the patient should he find that his needs are ignored, misunderstood, or not taken care of in the way he would prefer.

It is most important that, with one of these patients, the nurse convey her competence not only in words but also by concrete action. Thus, when she and her assistants lift him into his bath, they will do this in a way that will not cause him unnecessary additional pain, nor will it cause him to fear that they will drop him before he reaches his destination. The nurse also needs to convey to him, again more by her manner than in so many words, that she has some idea of what he might be going through. If there is reasonable assurance that there will be an improvement in the patient's state, the nurse should remind him of this fact on frequent occasions. As soon as she has some evidence that his initial panic has subsided—a change in the look in his eyes, his facial expression, or the color of his skin, perhaps—the nurse needs to work out with him the "Yes" and "No" arrangements we talked about in the preceding chapter.

In addition, the nurse needs to watch herself that she does not come to take the patient's handicap for granted. After all, at least certain states of immobilization of emotional or physical origin may gradually subside. Yet, if the patient finds himself confronted by an all-giving mother figure he may, for fear of hurting her feelings and thus arousing her anger and possible retaliation, renounce his slowly reemerging abilities to care for himself.

The resigned patient. There is another group of patients whose being overwhelmed by their conditions is expressed in an entirely different form. These patients are conscious and able to respond to what is happening to them. But they have given up all hope of gaining any kind of satisfaction from life, even though, at the present time at least, they may not be seriously incapacitated by their diseases. One finds this phenomenon frequently among patients who suffer from one or the other kind of cancerous condition (1). According to some theories, the cancer is not the cause of their pessimistic outlook but may rather be the result of a long-standing attitude of resignation on their part (2, 3, 4).

Whichever the case, the nurse frequently finds herself quite impatient with such clients. She feels that the patient still has a great deal to live for and is not utilizing to his best advantage the time still allocated to him. So she attempts to cheer him up and encourages him to participate in social activities and to take a more active interest in the affairs of the world. In her daily contacts with the patient she tries to indicate to him by an optimistic, brisk manner that all is not lost and that much could still be gained by him, if only he would make the necessary effort.

This is just the point, however; he cannot or does not want to make this effort. He feels that the nurse's frequent encouragements are an added load upon him imposed by an already hostile world that he does not have the energy or the interest to cope with.

To be of help to this kind of patient, the nurse must recognize that just by virtue of his attitude which manifests itself in a verbally or nonverbally expressed "Oh, what's the use," he is different from the one discussed above who seems to be "marooned in his immobilization" and who has to be literally coerced into becoming mobilized again. The resigned patient is not necessarily immobilized. He just does not have the energy it takes to move. If the nurse forces him into activity, he is likely to squander the little bit of energy he does have either by defending himself against her efforts or by going through with something he really does not care to do.

It would be better if the nurse were to respect the patient's resigned attitude as something which is deeply imbedded in his personality at this time, regardless of whether she believes that he has always been this way or that it is a result of his condition. Therefore, she will refrain from making any undue demands on his energy and instead unobtrusively offer him her quiet warmth. Slowly, she may be able to establish a bond with him. Or, perhaps she can be instrumental in fostering existing relationships he has, through helping the other persons to understand his limited ability to invest himself emotionally at this time.

Perhaps, slowly, the patient will become able to absorb energy from this warmth around him, just as one might absorb warmth from sitting, wrapped in blankets, in the noon sun on a fair, but cold fall day. He may then begin to show more interest in other matters of possible concern to him. The nurse should be careful, however, not to be too optimistic about his seeming spurt of energy, and should not egg him on into an ever-increasing cycle of activities. His organism has undoubtedly become attuned to a low energy level and is not equipped to handle a sudden increase in potential for very long (5). By being too active and too outgoing, the patient may exhaust his limited resources and may, sooner or later, have to fall back to an energy level which may be even lower than the one from which he started out.

The patient whose self-image is threatened. What about the patient who, although not too badly incapacitated by his condition at the moment, is terrified by the implications it is likely to have for his future or by the threat it represents to his cherished image of himself? Logically, patients in either of these two groups do not need to be unduly concerned about their situations. After all, they do not suffer acutely from their conditions, themselves, at the moment, and they may have ample time and means to adjust to the implications that they hold for the future. But is a patient likely to use logic when he finds out that he has Parkinson's disease, especially if he has had occasion to see what it does to a person as it advances, or if he has had opportunity to read about the likelihood of its being cured? And who could expect an otherwise healthy violinist not to feel that the loss of the use of his hand is tantamount to, or even worse than, the loss of his life would be?

It is particularly important that the nurse give these kinds of patients time to adjust to what has happened to them without pressuring them in that direction. They need a period during which they are permitted to withdraw their energies from the periphery so that they can take in what has happened to them and can realign themselves with it. Therefore, even though these patients are perhaps not quite as helpless as some of the other patients we have discussed, they too must be treated as if they actually could not help themselves. At the same time, the nurse needs to be alert to signs of the patient's moving from a stage of being overwhelmed by his condition to stages of beginning and increasing acceptance of it, and to give him the support he needs in each of these stages. How she will go about this has been discussed in Chapter 8 and elsewhere (6, 7, 8), and will be referred to again later on in this chapter.

He tries to escape awareness of his condition

By denial. Included in the group of patients who protect themselves from conscious awareness of their condition by irrational mechanisms of escape are, first of all, those who *deny* the existence of their conditions, in spite of objective evidence to the contrary. The young man who has just been fitted with a prosthesis and who walks on it for hours as if it were his own leg, completely oblivious to the pain this may cause him, and to the stump inflammation which is likely to result from it, is an example of this type of patient. So is the patient who, although he has once suffered a heart attack, treats his second attack as if it were a slight case of indigestion and who, for as long as he can, goes on with his life as if nothing had happened.

By transformation. Other patients not only deny their conditions' existence but transform them, in their minds, into their opposites. This is what happens, for instance, when a woman who has to undergo a hysterectomy not only denies the reality of her operation but is, in addition, convinced of the fact that she is with child.

By externalizing it. Then there is the patient who, although subliminally aware of what is happening to him, perceives it as if it were happening elsewhere, outside of himself. This phenomenon can often be observed in the patient who is in the process of undergoing a schizophrenic breakdown. He realizes that something is terribly wrong, but he is unable to conceive of the fact that it is his own personality that is crumbling. Instead, he may "know" that the world around him is about to collapse and he may beg his fellowmen to save themselves before it is too late.

By running away. Finally, there is the patient who, instead of consciously acknowledging his condition, figuratively or literally runs away from it. This kind of reaction can manifest itself, for example in a woman who has just found out that she has carcinoma of the breast, by an extreme state of overactivity that may closely resemble a manic episode. It may also manifest itself by a state of fugue in which a person suddenly finds himself at the other end of the continent without recollection as to how and why he got there.

Implications for nursing. In spite of the different ways that patients in this group may defend themselves against awareness of their conditions, there are certain common elements that have implications for nurses. First, the nurse needs to keep in mind that it will not do to reason with such a patient, for if he could listen to reason he would not have to act the way he does. Although he is experiencing his condition on some level, he is not able to confront it with his conscious mind. He cannot be held responsible, therefore, or blamed for his behavior toward his condition. At the same time, he must be protected, as far as possible, from the noxious effects that his attitude and behavior might bring about. That is, he should be kept in a protected environment and under sufficiently close surveillance that he has no way of hurting himself more than he is hurt already. This cannot always be done, however, for although irrational in some ways, these patients may not offer sufficient grounds for compulsory hospitalization. A man who states that his doctor has received the wrong laboratory results and therefore considers him to be a diabetic, cannot be put into an institution for saying this; nor can a woman who is told that before too long she will go blind because of a retinal detachment, very well be stopped from going on a spending spree. Sometimes, then, the nurse may have to stand by helplessly and observe the patient hurt himself and his loved ones. It may help her and the patient's family, perhaps, if they can come to understand that the impact of the realization of his condition might be more destructive for this particular patient than the effects of the condition per se.

How, then, should the nurse comport herself toward this patient? Should she go along with his escape mechanisms since he needs them to protect himself? I do not think so. True, she needs to accept and, perhaps, even to acknowledge to him his way of reacting to his state. Yet, at the same time she must get across to him that, as a health professional, she has a job to do which is spelled out for her via the physician's diagnosis and prescription, and by virtue of the patient's actions. Whether she will actually name the patient's condition or not will depend on how his physician would like the matter to be handled. Even if she does not attribute a label to his state, the nurse will need to be quite explicit and firm as to what the doctor's orders are and as to the fact that both she and the patient, while he is under her care, will have to comply with them. It will help, however, if, at the same time, the nurse can make herself available to the patient should he want to talk to her about what has happened to him. Perhaps, by using her as a sounding board, he can slowly, at his own rate, allow the meaning of what this is all about to penetrate into his awareness. The nurse must be especially careful, however, not to try to hurry this process; otherwise, the patient will become frightened and will have to retreat from it.

He refuses to accept his condition

Some patients, although consciously aware of their conditions, are either unable or unwilling to accept their states. Often they are terrified by what they think or know about their conditions. Because they fear their suspicions might be confirmed, they shy away from medical assistance. Most nurses have come across a patient with advanced metastatic cancer who had been aware for a long time that he had a tumor, but who was afraid of finding out that it was malignant, and had neglected to seek medical advice until he had to be admitted to the hospital for some unrelated, acute condition.

He fears knowing the truth. Usually, the patient's fear of finding out the truth about his condition does not manifest itself overtly. That is, the patient probably does not confide in anyone for fear that person might force him into taking the action that he is trying not to take. His terror may manifest itself, though, in other ways. Sometimes, a person of usually cheerful and outgoing disposition will become moody, irritable and withdrawn.

If asked what is the matter or if there is anything one can do for him, he will probably either gruffly or pleadingly demand that he be left alone.

Sometimes, because of his constant state of uncertainty and his anxiety about it, he may find it very difficult to concentrate on his job. Or, because he is depressed about what he thinks his condition to be, he may find that he is much too slow in everything he attempts to do. He might also find it increasingly difficult, therefore, to get out of bed in the morning and to stay up until his usual bed time.

He defies his condition. There is another group of patients who know what is the matter with them but who openly and willfully defy their conditions. They behave quite similarly to the ones who use denial as a mechanism of escaping the truth, but they know what they are doing while the others act without conscious intent. And so, one of these patients, even though fully aware of the fact that he has a serious kidney condition, and even though he has full knowledge of the stringent diet prescribed for him and the reasons for this diet, may well say to himself and to others, "To hell with it" and order a steak dinner and a big glass of beer.

He prefers to die. This group also includes the patient who, rather than going through with the suffering that he knows lies ahead of him, prefers to end his existence right then and there. He may be afraid that the pain will be too much for him and that he will not be able to bear it like a man. He may be afraid of the effects of his condition upon his appearance, his ability to perform, or his dignity as a human being. Therefore, he has decided to take his life in his own hands, at a time when he feels he is still in command of his reasoning power and still has the courage to go through with it.

He wants to undo past events. There are many other patients who, although quite aware of their condition, still do not want to accept the fact that it is true. They try to undo what has happened by dwelling upon what would have occurred if they or someone else had taken a different course of action at a certain time. These patients can be recognized by their frequent use of such statements as, "If only I had gone to the doctor for my yearly checkup," or "If only my husband had insisted that another doctor operate on me," or "Had I used his car, as he told me to, the accident would not have happened." This kind of rumination is one way of trying to keep the full impact of one's experience out of one's conscious awareness. However, since the flow of time is unfortunately irreversible, except in fiction, this way of defending himself against his experience is not going to be very useful to the patient in the long run.

He feels victimized. Finally, there is the patient who, although realizing that he is, for the time being, stuck with his condition, is very much put out by the fact that it should have befallen him, of all people. He not only lets you know that he suffers, but also how unfair it is that it should be he who is suffering so much. Of course, this is also a method that the patient uses to protect himself from having to integrate fully what has happened to him. Yet, as long as he resents having been "chosen," this patient, although accepting the treatment prescribed for him, is not likely to be willing to make the best of his life, in spite of his predicament.

Implications for nursing. Apart from caring for a patient in this group, what else can the nurse do to help him over the hump so that he can either get the medical help he needs or make the necessary peace with his state in order to integrate it constructively into his life? One way the nurse can be helpful to these patients is to make herself available to them should they wish to talk to her about how their conditions are affecting them. It will be helpful, also, if she acknowledges to each individual patient that she has some understanding of the way he feels as he does about his actual or anticipated state. In addition, she should try to expose the patient to the idea that there are both existing and potential resources within and outside himself. Hopefully, she can help him to assess his condition or his plans for dealing with it in light of these resources. That should be possible with a patient in this group, because he has already acknowledged the existence of his condition. It would be premature to use this approach with a patient who must escape from this realization (category two) and futile for the patient who is so overwhelmed by his condition (category one) that he is unable to mobilize his own resources or seek outside help.

Perhaps further discussion will illustrate this point more clearly. Suppose that among a public health nurse's case load there is a woman who confides in the nurse that she has been aware of a lump in her breast for several weeks. The moment the nurse suggests that she make an appointment with her physician, however, the patient becomes visibly frightened and switches to another topic. This behavior naturally puts the nurse in a very difficult position, for, on one hand, she has an obligation to help the patient seek care before it is too late; on the other hand, she does not want to cause her anguish. Besides, what is she to do if the patient refuses to discuss the matter with her? One cannot blame her wishing the patient had not confided in her in the first place, since she is not able or willing to follow through on the nurse's suggestion. Well, one thing the nurse can do is to inquire whether she has told anyone else, and if so, whom. Then she might inquire about what happened when she did tell someone. It may be that the patient had told her husband, and that for reasons of his own, he had become extremely anxious about the matter. Or, it may be that he had indicated to her that he would not be able to tolerate the truth if it turned out to be what they both very much feared it might be. To protect her husband, the patient may have avoided taking action. Perhaps, in this case, the nurse could talk with both of them, and possibly she could help the husband to verbalize his fears. It may be that his fears are based on exaggeration or misunderstanding and, in this case, it may well be within the nurse's power to alleviate these fears to some extent through clarification. On the other hand, his fears may be based on psychological needs which lie much deeper than mere misconceptions. If so, the nurse may be able to explore with him the possibility of his confiding in someone with whom he would feel free to talk over this serious matter that needs to be dealt with right away.

It may be that the patient is afraid of what might happen to her children if she were hospitalized, operated upon, and perhaps grossly disfigured. In this case, the nurse will have to discuss with the patient the resources available to her and perhaps help her to contact agencies that provide domestic help in emergencies. Or she may be able to secure the aid of a social service agency which will help the patient make the necessary arrangements.

It may also be that the patient is afraid of what her illness might do to her relationship with her husband. Depending upon the rapport the nurse has established with this patient, and her own security and skill in the exploration of such matters, she may either try to find out if there is anyone with whom the patient can discuss her fears, or she may try to help the patient to talk them over with her. It is hoped that the nurse can convey to the patient the urgency of the need for action as well as the assurance of support for the duration of her need of it.

It may be, however, that, in spite of the nurse's valiant attempt to help the patient to face the necessity of action, and in spite of her reassurance that she and her family will not be without support during the difficult time to come, the patient is still reluctant to make any move. If this should happen, the nurse may have to tell the patient that she will need to share this information with the physician and that he will take it from there. Confidence of this nature may not be kept from the physician in charge of the case, regardless of the patient's feelings. It is likely, though, that rather than resenting the nurse's move, the patient will be relieved by it. Had she really wanted no action at all, she would not have confided in the nurse in the first place. Also, when the situation is handled this way, the onus for initiating action and thus, starting an inexorable sequence of events, no longer lies with the patient. It has been shifted to the nurse.

What about the patient who openly defies his condition? Much depends upon how often this occurs. Everyone, even a very sick patient, needs to blow off steam once in a while to make room for the suffering ahead of him. The patient knows what he is doing and realizes the consequences of his actions. Although it may mean additional work and anguish for those who care for him, he is the one who will have to suffer the consequences and he is usually prepared to pay the price. It seems to me that the less said about such incidents, the better.

It is another matter, however, if his refusal to accept his condition is the rule rather than the exception. In such a case, the patient must be given the opportunity, at repeated intervals, to ventilate his anger and frustration in words, without being admonished about the way he is feeling. Perhaps, after the first heat has subsided, the nurse can ask him whether there might be other ways in which he could express his aggravation; ways for which he may not have to pay as dearly in return. Hopefully, he and the nurse can, together, arrive at such alternate, less costly ways of relieving his anger as talking about it, writing it down, or discharging it, if possible, through muscular action.

The patient who would rather die than live with his condition will probably need stronger psychological and spiritual support than the nurse and the physician alone can provide for him. He may require the help of a psychiatrist or a religious advisor, or both. Hopefully, this additional support will help the patient to realize that he does have the inner resources and outside aid that would make it possible for him to cope with what lies ahead. Hopefully, too, he can be helped to realize further, that loss of mastery of his life is not necessarily synonymous with "the end" of life altogether, for there might be ways of approaching his future which could be of deep significance, since they offer perspectives that he had never thought about while he was well and active. Thus, he may be able to learn to observe what goes on around and within him instead of merely trying to control it; he may be able to learn to receive instead of giving, as was his previous custom. By confronting his suffering with courage, he may convey a most valuable message to both his family and his fellow patients on the ward (9).

Not every patient will be able to make use of the support and the suggestions offered him. For many people, the idea of what they will have to go through, and their inner conviction that they cannot and will not be able to bear it, is so powerful that they cannot even consider an alternative. In any case, the nurse has no right to let the patient end his life prematurely as long as he is under her care. This is one message she must not fail to communicate to him.

The patient who tries to alter the course of his own past history requires a great deal of patience from his nurse. His ruminations of "what would have happened, if only . . ." have become part of his life and are his answer to most everyday problems he encounters. And so, each time his bell is not answered, each time he is treated with less respect than he feels he is due, each time a tray of cold food that should be hot is set before him, he wishes that he had not signed the permission slip for the operation, or that he had gone to Dr. B. instead of Dr. A. Perhaps, in their discussions, the nurse can help him to accept the fact that he had not acted irresponsibly then, that he had used the best judgment available to him and that, had he made a different decision, he might not necessarily be much better off today. In addition, the nurse should try to help him to focus on what is going on now, what is really aggravating him, and what is within his power to change and what is not. Hopefully, he can, in time, derive satisfaction from the powers that he does have, and not become too upset about matters beyond his control. Here, much will depend upon the over-all quality of the care he is receiving. Unfortunately, there are many situations in which disrespect and neglect of the patient are as overwhelming as the lack of power on the part of himself and the nurse to alter things. In this case, the patient's ruminations may be the only means by which he can preserve his sanity.

The patient who feels sorry for himself because he has been

singled out to suffer this way may also need the additional support of a psychiatrist or of a religious advisor, provided he is willing to accept it. With this kind of patient, the nurse must be particularly careful that she does not judge him too harshly. His self-pity, his whining and frequent complaining about the way he has been treated by God, or by fate, may be a culturally prescribed way of behaving which need not necessarily reflect his personal convictions. Thus, how else is a woman from southern Italy or an older Jewish woman to let both her doctor and her family know that she is the patient? How else is she to let them know that she expects them to give her the supports that are also culturally prescribed, such as visiting her en masse not only in the hospital but also when she is convalescing at home, sending her cards and flowers, and seeing to it that her home continues to be taken care of, even though not quite as efficiently as when she was well? The patient's feeling sorry for himself may also be just an intermediate step in his learning to accept his condition. He will get over it in time.

Another patient may have certain ideas as to what he and his life should be like, and he is simply unable to revise these preconceptions. Naturally, his current state interferes with his self-view, so why should he not be filled with self-pity? The nurse could try to suggest the possibility that life and one's progress in it cannot be predicted with 100 per cent accuracy. In many instances, however, she will find that the patient becomes very anxious at the mention of such thoughts.

Perhaps, the nurse can help the patient to gain some satisfaction and enjoyment from capacities that have been left untouched by his illness or that have been brought into play because of it. I remember one patient in his early sixties who had a severe and progressive heart condition and was unable to leave his home and go to work. Whenever the public health nurse visited him, he would receive her with tears in his eyes, and an expression on his face which plainly said, "Look what has become of me." The nurse did not protest against his attitude, but she did not show much sympathy for it either. Instead, she asked to see what he had accomplished during the week since her last visit. His face lit up as he showed her two paintings he had started. One was a self-portrait and the other a view of his garden from his bedroom window. The nurse had not had much training in art, but she could tell from the composition and color of his paintings that his was a more than ordinary talent which was finally finding expression. From her previous visits, she knew that he had not touched a paintbrush once during the forty or more years since he had left school and had started to work as an engineer. Neither he nor the nurse voiced their thoughts, but both knew, and knew that the other knew that, in spite of what his condition had done to him and to his life, it also had its compensations.

He uses his condition for ulterior purposes

On accasion, we all take advantage of certain conditions we may have, and I think we should be permitted to do so for short periods of time now and then.

For a brief respite. Most of us enjoy the luxury of leaving work early because of a severe cold, perhaps, and of abdicating our responsibilities for the rest of the day. Most of us feel not only relief, but also a certain sense of gratification once we are in bed under warm blankets and are sipping a hot drink. We are also probably secretly pleased when the doctor orders us to stay in bed one more day because, under the sanction of medical authority, we may indulge ourselves in reading a mystery novel on a week-day, interrupted only by the arrival of our meals, brought to us on trays by our solicitous spouse, or a neighbor or friend.

So, let us not pass judgment on the patient who is able to derive a certain degree of satisfaction from letting others take care of him; let us rather help him enjoy his dependent state. A small amount of "secondary gain," as this phenomenon is called, will not hurt the patient or those who take care of him. On the contrary, it can provide a certain reserve of well-being for him to fall back on later when he is again trying to maintain his footing in the mainstream of a busy life.

To avoid solving problems. There are other ways of using one's condition that are less harmless than the one just described. For instance, the patient who lacks skill in problem-solving or in relating to others may become ill whenever he does not know how to cope with a situation or whenever communication with others becomes strained. Often, while he is out of circulation, the problem resolves itself. Consequently, the patient is not likely to be any better prepared for the next hurdle he encounters and may, therefore, have to resort to illness over and over again. The chances are that the price he must pay for this will sooner or later entail loss of income, loss of his job and, probably, eventual loss of patience by all those who associate with him.

To avoid disturbing the family equilibrium. Nurses who work in the field of mental health frequently encounter patients who choose to be ill in order to maintain the delicate equilibrium that exists in their families or in a family member. These patients say, and know from past experience, that when their health improves, the health of the mother or another member of the family will invariably deteriorate. These patients voluntarily shoulder the sick role, and all the hardships that go with it, in order to protect the other person, whom they consider to be less endowed with strength.

I remember one patient who, because of a birth defect, was somewhat retarded and also had some difficulty with muscular coordination. For 45 years, this man allowed his mother to take care of his most intimate personal and bodily needs in order "not to upset" her. Then his mother died and, surprisingly, with very little practice, this patient learned to bathe, dress, shave himself and take care of his elimination unaided, and to do such other things for himself as cutting his own meat at meals. I must add, however, that often in such cases the newly won independence can go to the patient's head to such an extent that he does not adhere to any rules or regulations. He may become so active, and full of projects at all hours of the day and night, that his indomitable energies create serious problems for the personnel of an institution.

Some patients feel compelled to enact the role of black sheep, with whatever meaning this may have for a particular family. Other family members deposit their blackness on him and are thus enabled to appear white and hence, acceptable to themselves and to each other. The nurse in the mental health field knows what would happen to the precarious state of health of these family members if the patient should learn to differentiate between his own black aspects and those which are not his, and if he should refuse to accept the latter.

To hold power over others. A third group of patients are those who use their condition as a means of gaining or maintaining power over other people. We have all heard of a mother or father who announced an impending heart attack upon hearing that one of the children in the family was attracted to a member of the opposite sex. If this did not prove an effective deterrant to continuation of the affair, the parent actually collapsed on or just before the wedding day. Many of us have known patients who threatened to go into a convulsion, and did not hesitate to follow through on this threat, when requests for extra privileges were not immediately considered and approved. Then there is the patient who is able to use his own fear of crowds, bridges or tunnels to keep a solicitous spouse safely at home with him, away from the dangerous influence of others. Finally, patients who are liable to have asthmatic attacks at the slightest provocation, are often spared—by their loved ones—the aggravation and effort entailed in assuming responsibilities or making decisions.

To gain prestige. One other group of patients belonging to the category of those who use their conditions for ulterior purposes are those who are proud of their conditions and consider them accomplishments. In mild form, this phenomenon is not only harmless but serves as an innocent recompense for having to undergo painful periods in one's life. Frequently, during conversations in waiting rooms of doctor's offices or clinics, or large hospital wards, each patient will attempt to gain prestige in the eyes of the others by trying to excel in the number or severity of operations he has had to undergo, the size and amount of stones found in his kidney or gall bladder, or the quantity of drainage tapped from his peritoneal cavity. This bragging, macabre as it may be, constitutes only one aspect of these patients' lives, however. Almost without exception, they will later resume their normal life roles, albeit with a touch of heroism from now on.

To obtain self-worth. For some patients, the only way to find self-worth, and thus possible worth in the eyes of others, seems to lie in their taking frequent trips to the operating room. They apparently possess little else in life than their ailments and a need to have these looked into with the aid of a surgeon. Nurses who have come across such patients in their work experience may find such encounters quite disturbing, for there is something eerie and frightening about the way these patients almost gleefully submit themselves to one operation after another, apparently without fear of the accompanying pain or the outcome. The only thing that seems to give them satisfaction is to add to their already numerous scars which they are proud to exhibit. These people are apparently oblivious to what their illnesses might mean to their families. They take it for granted that they are the center of their families' attention and feel no obligation to show any concern for them in return. I suppose their lack of feeling toward those close to them can only be understood in light of the deep-lying lack of affection for themselves which exhibits itself by this punitive attitude toward their bodies.

Implications for nursing. Can we derive a general principle of nursing care that might be valid for all patients belonging in this category? Every one of these patients who uses his illness for ulterior purposes, regardless of whether he is indulging in a benign pastime or is exhibiting a serious lack of preparation for life is, consciously or unconsciously, either deriving or dispensing a certain amount of benefit from his actions. Therefore, it would not be fair for the nurse to ask him to stop what he is doing, especially when the patient, himself, is not aware of his goals.

I think that we can safely go along with the patient who enjoys the secondary gains of a brief illness or the one who is proud of the fact that his fractured bone had to be reset four times as against only three resettings of his neighbor's.

Patients who have no skill in coping with their life problems and need to use their conditions for this purpose will have to be allowed to use this outlet until they acquire sufficient skill in living to do otherwise. In order to acquire such skill, they must, as a first step, admit their lack of it. This is a difficult thing to do; it is especially difficult for adults of whom a certain amount of proficiency in living is expected. Therefore, it is imperative for the nurse to establish a relationship with the patient in which he can, after a time, feel safe to expose his lack of proficiency to her and ask for guidance. To do this, the nurse must refrain from being judgmental of the patient, even when his lack of skill seems rather inappropriate for someone of his age. In addition, it will help if the nurse can project herself as a person who is not uncomfortable in the knowledge that she is by no means perfect, but who keeps learning from her mistakes and does not expect to be all-knowing or infallible. Slowly, as the patient acquires and tests out new skills in living, his need to be ill will occur less and less frequently.

What about the patient who tries to shoulder responsibility for the destiny of his entire family? Usually, he will need expert professional help in addition to that which the nurse can give. He will have to learn, slowly, and with the help of a trusting relationship to another human being who does not exploit him (as his family probably has done), that each person is—ultimately—an entity unto himself. True, each individual in our society is expected to take the responsibility of raising his children according to his best judgment and, in most cultures, is also expected to take responsibility for the care of his aged, ailing or financially dependent relatives. This does not mean, however, that one must sacrifice one's uniqueness (which includes one's limitations as to how much one has to give to others) in order to spare these others the travail of having to cope with life in their unique ways. On the contrary, when one does take on this responsibility, he sets himself up as more powerful than anyone has the right to be. Also, by blurring the lines of demarcation between himself and others, he makes it much more difficult for the others to work out their own destinies. But should this person's mother, or brother, or wife become ill as his own health begins to improve, would he then not be guilty of having caused the illness? Yes, in a way, but only in the way that any person who begins to realize his own potential is guilty of offending those who, for reasons of their own, cannot tolerate this change. The anxiety arising from this guilt is one he will need to learn to live with. This will be easier for him to do if he can view it as an opportunity for his loved ones to test their own potentials and strengths.

The patient who, consciously or unconsciously, utilizes his condition to control those around him will also need expert help in addition to that of the nurse. This patient is, in a way, not sufficiently differentiated from his close relatives; rather, they are part of him, as it were, and he feels that he cannot let them be on their own because this would deprive him of a large part of himself. One way of helping him is to let him identify the "indispensables" in his loved ones, i.e., those qualities in the others without which he feels he cannot exist. Once the patient has identified these qualities in another, he can be asked whether, perhaps, he, too, possesses similar qualities, for we usually cherish in others that which is also present, although not always recognized, in ourselves. With support and concrete guidance, the patient can gradually learn to know, love, and develop his own qualities and, eventually, he may be able to relinquish the other person to his own life without necessarily disrupting the relationship between them and also without having to undergo a serious health crisis because of it. Because this is a slow process, and the rewards are slow in coming, it may not appeal to every patient belonging to this group. When the patient is not inclined to accept the help offered him, the nurse may find that she can use her energies to good effect in lending support to those family members who also need to find themselves but are afraid of doing so because of the health crises this may provoke in the patient.

The patient who seemingly lives for the sole purpose of undergoing surgery repeatedly presents a very difficult problem for the nurse. She finds it awkward, and rightly so, to give him the recognition he craves on the only basis on which he asks for it, i.e., the progressive mutilation of his body. In addition, this patient tends to be very unappreciative of what the nurse does for him and thereby puts the nurse even more on the defensive. Perhaps it will help the nurse to realize that this patient (it is usually a woman) really has no feeling of warmth, for herself or for others. It may further help the nurse to try to get some idea of why this patient must be the way she is instead of disapproving of her actions. Probably the most meaningful explanation she will find is that the patient had been deprived in a very cruel way during her childhood, although not everyone who has been so deprived needs to be as cruel to himself and his family as this patient is. Perhaps, keeping her mind open for clues that might help her understand the patient, coupled with a certain amount of unconditional warmth, will keep the nurse on safe footing for the duration of the patient's stay. The chances are that this patient will not represent a success story for her, neither now nor when she returns for more surgery. On the other hand, just because she presents such an enigma to the nurse, she might be considered a challenge in whom the nurse could profitably invest her energy.

He accepts his condition for what it is

The fifth category of interrelationships between patient's conditions and their experiences is the acceptance of his condition by the patient; that is, he is able to make the best of his life in spite of his illness, without having to complain about it, without needing to resent it and without capitalizing on it. This does not happen very often, nor does it happen over night. Most patients, even those who are eventually able to reach this stage of acceptance, will probably have to struggle through a number of phases, some of which were mentioned earlier in this chapter and have also been described by other authors (10, 11). Even after the stage of acceptance has been reached, it is not necessarily a constant state. When the odds against the patient are too great, or when he suffers excruciating pain or profound humiliation, for instance, he may well have to revert, for a time at least, to less mature ways of coping with his state. The nurse should not hold it against him that he must slip back once in a while.

Often it is not so much a matter of accepting one's condition as realizing and accepting one's tendency toward it. Once the condition has developed fully, it may take hold of the patient to such an extent that there is little he can do about it while it lasts. This is true for many illnesses, including malaria, depression and even gall bladder attacks; it is also true for the impulsive behavior, irritability and compulsive habits discussed in Chapter 10. In other words, the condition is always there, latent or lurking in the background, ready to take over the patient's organism if he submits to more stress than he can handle or to the particular stress which is likely to provoke his ailment. A patient who is able to accept his tendency toward a certain condition will try to avoid extremes of mental, physical and emotional exertion, and to avoid situations or actions that he knows, from past experience, bring the condition into the open. If he cannot do so, for inner or outer reasons beyond his control, he will at least try to seek help as soon as he feels his condition coming upon him, before it takes over his powers of judgment, causes him to act in ways that he may have to regret later on, or possibly, overwhelms him altogether.

Ideally, a nurse should be able to help each of her patients to reach the state of acceptance of his condition. In practice, she may not be able to do this very often, because the severity and nature of the patients' condition, the lack of time they have to work on the problem together, the patient's lack of ability and willingness to be helped, and the nurse's lack of skill in helping him are all factors that may well interfere, either alone or jointly, in the process. This interference need not necessarily be paralyzing to the nurse, however. She can start with what she has to offer and learn from each new experience. As long as she appropriately applies her knowledge to the patient in his current state, she helps to initiate a process that, even if not visible at first, may well continue in the right direction even after she and the patient have parted ways.

References

1. Bahnson, Claus Bahne. "Emotional Reactions to Internally and Externally Derived Threat to Annihilation" in *The Threat of Impending Disaster* (George Grosser *et al.*, eds.). Cambridge, Mass.: M.I.T. Press, 1964.
2. Reich, Wilhelm. *Selected Writings*. New York: Farrar, Straus, 1960.
3. LeShan, L. "An Emotional Life History Pattern Associated with Neoplastic Disease." A paper presented at a conference on the psychophysical aspects of cancer. The New York Academy of Sciences, April, 1965.
4. Schmale, Arthur H., and Iker, Howard P. "The Psychological Setting of Uterine Cervical Cancer." A paper presented at a conference on psychophysiological aspects of cancer. The New York Academy of Sciences, April, 1965.
5. Reich, Wilhelm. *Op. cit.*
6. Ujhely, Gertrud B. "Basic Considerations for Nurse-Patient Interaction in the Prevention and Treatment of Emotional Disorders," *Nursing Clinics of North America 1*:2 (June, 1966), pp. 179-186.
7. Ujhely, Gertrud G. "Grief and Depression—Implications for Preventive and Therapeutic Nursing Care," *Nursing Forum* 5:2, 1966, pp. 23-35.
8. Ujhely, Gertrud B. *The Nurse and Her Problem Patients*. Springer Publishing Co., 1963.

9. Frankl, Viktor E. "Fragments from the Logotherapeutic Treatment of Four Cases" in *Modern Psychotherapeutic Practice* (Arthur Burton, ed.). Palo Alto, Calif.: Science and Behavior Books, 1966.
10. Lederer, Henry D. "How the Sick View Their World" in *Patients, Physicians and Illness* (E. Gartley Jaco, ed.). Glencoe, Ill.: The Free Press, 1958.
11. Engel, George L. *Psychological Development in Health and Disease*. Philadelphia: W. B. Saunders Co., 1962.

Suggested Readings

Glasser, William. *Reality Therapy*. New York: Harper, 1965.

Green, Hannah. *I Never Promised You a Rose Garden*. New York: Holt, Reinhart and Winston, 1964.

Hacket, Thomas, and Weisman, Avery T. "Reactions to the Imminence of Death" in *The Threat of Impending Disaster* (George Grosser *et al.*, eds.). Cambridge, Mass.: M.I.T. Press, 1964.

Harding, M. Esther. *The "I" and the "Not-I."* Princeton, N. J.: Princeton University Press, 1965.

Hodgins, Eric. *Episode: Report on the Accident Inside My Skull*. New York: Atheneum, 1964.

Jung, Carl G. "Two Essays in Analytical Psychology" in *Collected Works, VII*. New York: Pantheon Books, 1953.

Kluckhohn, Florence R. "Variations in the Basic Values of Family Systems" in *A Modern Introduction to the Family* (Norman Bell and Ezra F. Vogel, eds.). Glencoe, Ill.: The Free Press, 1960.

Menninger, Karl *et al. The Vital Balance*. New York: Viking Press, 1963.

Poole, P. E. "Implementing Behavior in Male Patients with Coronary Artery Disease," *Nursing Research 15* (Spring, 1966), pp. 172-174.

Priestley, J. B. "Time and the Conveys" in *Seven Plays*. New York: Harper and Bros., 1950.

Ruesch, Juergen. *Disturbed Communication*. New York: W. W. Norton & Co., 1957.

Searles, Harold F. *Collected Papers on Schizophrenia and Related Subjects*. New York: International Universities Press, 1965.

Spiegel, John. "Cultural Variations in Attitudes Toward Death and Disease" in *The Threat of Impending Disaster* (George Grosser *et al.*, eds.). Cambridge, Mass.: M.I.T. Press, 1964.

Stone, Alan A., and Stone, Sue Smart. *The Abnormal Personality Through Literature*. Englewood Cliffs, N. J.: Prentice-Hall, 1966.

Tillich, Paul. *The Courage to Be*. New Haven, Conn.: Yale University Press, 1952.

Wickes, Frances G. *The Inner World of Childhood* (2nd ed.). New York: Appleton-Century-Crofts, 1966.

Wickes, Frances G. *The Inner World of Choice*. New York: Harper, 1963.

Wickes, Frances G. *The Inner World of Man*. New York: Frederick Ungar Publishing Co., 1959.

Zborowski, Mark. "Cultural Components in Responses to Pain" in *Patients, Physicians and Illness* (E. Gartley Jaco, ed.). Glencoe, Ill.: The Free Press, 1958.

Chapter 12

The Patient's Physical and Behavioral Self

Nurses are often called upon to take care of patients whose diagnoses have not yet been established and whose capacities for experience, or lack of it, cannot be ascertained at first sight. These are frequently newly admitted patients, some of whom may come under the nurse's care even before they have been seen by a physician and thus there are no doctor's orders to guide her approach. Sometimes they are patients who have developed another condition or complications during the course of their original illnesses.

To be of help to such a patient the nurse will need to look for clues other than the ones we have discussed so far. She will have to call on her experience and her knowledge, along with her ability to utilize consciously her powers of perception, interpretation and response.

Assessing the Patient's Condition and Needs

Suppose a newly admitted patient is brought to the ward. He is sitting in a wheelchair as is the custom in many hospitals. The slip accompanying the patient says "For observation." This does not tell the nurse very much about his condition. At first glance, however, she notes that he is somewhat cyanotic around the nose and mouth, and that his fingernails are also bluish rather than pink. The nurse greets the patient by name, introduces herself and states that she is the staff nurse on this section of the ward. As the patient answers her greeting, she notices that his voice is somewhat hoarse and that his breathing is labored. She notices also that, after speaking those few words, he started to cough—a harsh, unproductive cough. As she wheels him toward his room, the nurse reflects upon the probability that he is suffering from some kind of condition that interferes with his oxygen intake. She has no way of knowing, of course, whether this may be due primarily to malfunctioning of his heart, his lungs or his larynx. Whatever the cause of his respiratory difficulties, she knows that it will probably help the patient if the head end of his bed is raised somewhat; how far it should be raised will be up to him to determine. She also knows that, for the time being at least, it will be wise for her not to engage him in lengthy conversations. She knows further that this patient needs not only fresh air but warmth, especially for his lower extremities which, although she has not seen them without their coverings, she expects to be at least as poorly supplied with oxygen and as cyanotic as are his hands and nose.

After helping the patient out of his wheelchair, showing him his room and making sure that his call bell is in good working order and that he knows how to use it, the nurse asks him whether he feels able to undress himself or whether he would like to have assistance. The patient states that he has been taking care of himself all along. The nurse decides that allowing him to do this one more time, until specific orders from the physician are available, will not harm the patient too much and may save him unnecessary embarrassment. Before she leaves the room, however, she fluffs the pillows, raises the head end of the bed about thirty degrees, loosens the bed-clothes at the foot end, and checks whether there is enough heat coming from the radiator. She asks the patient to ring for her as soon as he is in bed, and promises that when she returns she will have an additional blanket for his feet, will open the window and adjust the head end of his bed to his liking, and will be able to tell him when he can expect to see his physician.

On her way to the nurses' station she looks once more at the admission slip. Joseph Schneiderhahn, age 45. Probably of German extraction, she thinks. Yet, in the few words he had exchanged with her, the nurse had not distinguished the slightest trace of accent. He must have been born in this country or perhaps he came here when he was still a little boy. On the other hand the "sch" in his name points to the possibility that he may still adhere to certain old-world values, particular to his country of origin, such as punctuality, order, cleanliness and, perhaps also a certain literalness with respect to the giving and taking of messages. All of these suppositions remain to be verified, however, after she has had more opportunity to get to know the patient.

The nurse's thoughts also dwell for a moment on the image the patient had left in her mind after she had helped him out of the chair and had walked with him to the bathroom and then back to his bed. He is of short, stocky build and gives the impression of having had ample opportunity to develop the muscles of his arms and chest. He must have spent much of his life in athletics or doing physical labor—probably the latter, she thinks, for when he took the call bell in his hand, she noticed that he held it gingerly as though used to handling large, bulky objects rather than small and relatively fragile ones. Also, the nurse noted that the palms of his hands were thick-skinned and callused and that his fingernails, though clean, were bruised here and there. She must be careful not to use highfalutin language with him until she has a better idea as to what his level of education might be. There were brown stains on his fingers, probably from nicotine, but in light of his respiratory difficulty, she has decided against offering him an ash tray unless he specifically asks for it.

She is glad that the admission slip mentioned the patient's age. His rather weather beaten face and neck would have made it hard for her to judge whether he might be nearer forty or fifty. The nurse hopes, for his sake and that of his family (is he married? does he have small children?), that he does not have emphysema, or a malignant tumor in his lung or larynx, or a poorly compensated heart defect.

Although he had seemed somewhat ill at ease, the patient had not appeared overly frightened by his admission to the hospital. The nurse realizes however, that his composure may merely have been a reflection of the way he usually deals with stressful situations. She makes a mental note to give him a chance to ask her questions when she returns to his room, so that he can at least have some answers about such easily explained matters as routine procedures, visiting hours, the location of phones, and the availability of newspapers and magazines.

We can see from this example that by being consciously aware of the impressions conveyed to her by her sensory organs, and by linking these observations to her store of knowledge, the nurse has been able to gain quite a bit of preliminary information from which she can derive tentative guidelines for her interaction with the patient. Of course, these guidelines are subject to confirmation or revision in light of further observation, validation from the patient, and additional information gathered from him, his physician and other sources, including the aide assigned to answer his bell. The greater the nurse's observational skills and the more extensive her knowledge, the more meaningful will be the tentative conclusions she can draw; the greater her willingness to revise her conclusions in light of additional information, the greater the chance that she will be able to render appropriate and individualized care.

The nurse took many factors into account when trying to make a tentative assessment of the patient and his needs for nursing care. Several of these factors have already been discussed at length, although in a different context, in Part I. Therefore, we shall deal with them only briefly here.

Factors That Influence the Nurse-Patient Relationship

Age

One very important factor the nurse always has to consider is the patient's age. Knowing how old he is can shed some light on the kind of condition he might have. It can also guide the nurse as to how she should formulate her messages to him so that he may be able to receive, understand and process them. For example, an infant cannot be assured by verbal promises that everything is going to be all right. It is able, however, to be influenced by the tone of the message and by its translation into concrete action. Thus, an infant will respond favorably to a soft voice and to gentle hands that hold it securely so that it need not fear it will fall. It will also be likely to respond with increasing trust when it finds out that its cries of discomfort are heeded and that it is changed and fed in accordance with its own rhythm rather than with that of a clock.

Similarly, remembering that preschoolers do not see time entities in the same way adults do, the nurse refrains from telling a toddler that his mother will be back in "three hours" or "at two o'clock." Instead, she will say that his mother will be back "after lunch" or after he "has had his nap."

By finding out from his parents what words the child uses for meals, elimination, sleep and pain, and using them, the nurse can forestall a great deal of anxiety that might otherwise develop. Frequently a child may become tense or cry when he is hungry or tired, when he needs to urinate or defecate or when he suffers pain. Although unable to translate his discomfort into the appropriate word by himself, if asked in his own vocabulary whether this or that is bothering him, he will probably recognize the term and respond appropriately. On the other hand, words with which he is not familiar, although they may denote the same thing to the nurse that the child's words do, may cause him to feel more distressed and even abandoned.

Small children may dislike having their bodies exposed in front of other children or adults of the opposite sex just as much as adults do. When a child clings frantically to his covers at the approach of a nurse or a physician, he may be more afraid of being exposed than of the contemplated procedure. It is important, therefore, that the nurse safeguard his modesty during medical examinations as well as when giving him a bath or an enema.

Some nurses confuse the facts that a child is not as yet capable of abstract thinking and that it responds more totally to stimuli than older people, with the notion that a child, if told that it will not feel pain will actually not feel it and, what is more, will not respond to it. Perhaps they would also like to protect the child from having to suffer in anticipation of the painful event and at the same time, protect themselves from having to listen to the vocal expression of his anticipatory suffering. But what happens to a child's feeling that adults are trustworthy if he is told that the incision of a boil, the suturing of a cut, or the setting of a fractured bone without anesthesia will not hurt at all? Is it not better to tell him the truth and also that the hurt will go away soon after the painful procedure is completed?

The two age ranges most difficult for many nurses to cope with are adolescence and senium. As we all know, adolescents are at an "awkward" age—an age the nurse would probably like to forget as far as her own behavior is concerned, or possibly one that she herself has barely outgrown. The adolescent is no longer a child, as is proved by his appearance, yet often he acts worse than a child in that he seems to intentionally provoke the nurse and to put her "on the spot." Whether it is his awkwardness with himself and others that makes the nurse uneasy with him or whether it is his uncanny skill in pointing to the "chip" she carries with dignity on her shoulder, she is frequently at a loss as to how to relate to him. If she treats him like a child, he is likely to rebel and make life even harder for her. If she acts more "professional," i.e., dignified, than she normally would, he is likely to laugh at her, either outright, or as she turns her back but still in time for her to notice it.

The more comfortable the nurse can be with her own shortcomings and the more she is able to see the adolescent as a young, though still inexperienced adult, the better she and he will get along. Also, the more she can keep some of the adolescent's idiosyncrasies in mind, the more competent the care she will be able to give. Thus, remembering that adolescents are very sensitive about their appearance, she will refrain from commenting on it unless asked about it first. If she has to give him direction or advice, she will be careful to transmit it in the form of a suggestion rather than an order. Instead of insisting upon being helpful to him, especially in areas where he can help himself, it will be better if she encourages the adolescent to be of assistance to others. Remembering, too, the adolescent's need for privacy, the nurse will make a special effort to respect it; for example she will remain with the female adolescent patient, whom she has draped carefully, during an examination performed by a professional member of the opposite sex; and she will excuse herself and leave the room when a male adolescent patient is being examined by his male physician.

On the whole, it seems that many nurses find patients who are in their own age group more attractive, but not necessarily easier to work with, than older or younger ones. It is more difficult to distinguish between one's professional and social roles when interacting with a potentially eligible member of the opposite sex than it is when interacting with someone forty years one's junior or senior. Also, the danger of identifying with the patient to the point of being so immersed in his problem that one loses one's ability to be of help, is also greater with a patient who, "but for the grace of God," could be oneself.

Nurses frequently treat older people in a condescending way without being aware of it and probably also without meaning any harm. Perhaps this has to do with the unenviable status of the aged in our society at large; perhaps the nurse merely means to be friendly because the patient reminds her of her own parent, grandparent, uncle or aunt. And so, a nurse may call an older patient whom she is seeing for the first time, "mom" or "pop." Or, because she expects him to have a certain hearing loss and also greater difficulty in finding his bearings in a new environment, she may unconsciously raise her voice far more than is necessary, and may order him around rather than offer suggestions as she would have done if he were younger.

It is not enough for the nurse to know that these are not appropriate ways of relating to older patients. She also needs to be constantly on guard against the temptation to treat them as if they were less intelligent and less competent than younger people and as if, because of deficits in sensory perception and slower pace, they were also lacking in sensitivity. By being aware of this temptation, the nurse has a better chance to defend herself against it than if she denies that it exists. A good way to keep from treating an older person as if he had outlived his usefulness is to find out, as soon as possible, more about the patient's background and his past and current interests and, if this is not contraindicated by his condition, to engage him in discussion about these things (*see* Chapter 8). This will bring the humanity of the person more into the foreground and will help to override the stereotyped view one tends to form of people in this age group.

Sociocultural background

Another important factor, or rather a cluster of factors, that the patient brings to his relationship with the nurse is his sociocultural background. In itself, the patient's origin should make no difference to the nurse, since she has sworn that she would care for him on the basis of his need, "with respect for human dignity, unrestricted by considerations of nationality, race, creed, color or status" (American Nurses' Association, *Code of Ethics*, 1960). However, since his background influences the way that the patient experiences and conceives of his condition, his patient role and his caretakers, and since it may influence the way his caretakers respond to him, it does make a great deal of difference and should be taken into serious consideration by the nurse.

At the same time, she needs to realize that people do not act in certain ways simply because they are Jewish, or Negro, or upper or lower class. These terms are merely shorthand expressions for a multitude of phenomena. A single word stands for an entire value system and mode of communication that has evolved over a long time and is still evolving, partly determined by and partly in response to the society in which a particular subgroup finds itself. For example, to be a "Christian" means something quite different today than it meant at the time of the Crusaders or in the second century of the Roman Empire. Similarly, to be a Negro means something quite different in Haiti than it does in South Africa. Also, the term "class" is a composite of several such important variables as the number of years one has gone to school and one's current occupation, each one of which influences the way a person looks at and communicates with his world. Often one variable will determine the others; for instance, because of one's race or religion, or the time his ancestors reached the country where he now resides, one may be permitted, by the dominant culture, to attain a certain class status, but not to go on to the next one above.

Whenever the nurse cares for a patient from a minority group, it will be helpful for her to realize that the longer a minority group resides in an area influenced by a dominant culture, the more of that culture's values it will absorb, including the way that it looks upon people of its own group. Sometimes, this results in a conflict of values that can literally paralyze a person or cause him to try to liberate himself from it by violent acts of defiance. Sometimes, it may spur him on to high creative effort, and to a search for peace with his own identity.

It will also be helpful for the nurse to gain increasing insight into the stresses that particular cultures, religions, classes and ethnic groups impose upon their members, and the effects these stresses may have on the genesis of her patient's condition as well as on the way he deals with it.

Whatever the combination of sociocultural variables the patient presents to the nurse, it will help her to remember that his way of reacting to his condition and to the hospital staff is probably just as right for him as her own way would be for her if she were the patient. The clearer she is concerning her own value system and her preferred way of communicating with others, and the more she knows about those sociocultural determinants that may cause the patient to act the way he does, the more chance she will have of understanding the patient's communications and of formulating her own message within a frame of reference that is understandable and acceptable to him.

The patient's sociocultural background, or the culture in which he presently finds himself, will also determine to a considerable degree the way a man or woman of a certain age will comport himself in various roles that link him to other people. The fact that in some cultural subgroups a son brings flowers to his ailing mother and visits her in the hospital every day for two hours does not necessarily mean that he loves his mother more dearly than does a son from a different background who sends his mother a sheer, sleeveless nightgown and lets her know via telephone that he is thinking of her. Similarly, parents who prefer that their children be seen but not heard may not love them any more or any less than those who find it natural that their 3- to 6-year-old children participate in their parents' conversations with other adults.

Signs and symptoms

Another group of phenomena that the patient brings to the relationship are the signs and symptoms that he exhibits. Although some of these manifestations are usually linked to the other factors we have discussed (i.e. the patient's experience, his condition, his socioeconomic background and his age), his signs and symptoms have to be considered by themselves; at times, when they are acute, they may override all other considerations. Thus, when a patient suddenly goes into shock or starts hemorrhaging, the nurse has to do everything in her power to counteract this physiological occurrence; she can be concerned only secondarily with whether she has properly explained all procedures to him or whether she has safeguarded his need for privacy. It would be infinitely more harmful to the patient if the nurse were to let considerations of his cultural background or his age override lifesaving actions than the other way around. If she is successful in the remedial measures that she initiates, such as lowering the head end of the patient's bed, covering him with a blanket, seeing to it that the physician is called and that emergency equipment (in good order) is available to him, the patient will be in a position to forgive her for lack of courtesy during the lifesaving procedures. If she follows an opposite course, he may not live to see the day when he can be unforgiving. Of course, the more skillful the nurse, the better she will be able to keep the patient's various facets in mind while at the same time working to overcome the danger to his life.

Not all signs and symptoms are of such acute nature, however. In fact, some of them are of such chronic prevalence that they form the main "bone of contention" between patient and nurse. Among the more common chronic symptoms are recurrent pain, lack of sleep, or the expressed need for mechanical respiratory aid as soon as the patient experiences the slightest twinge of uneasiness.

Pain. If pain is anticipated, the patient's physician leaves an order for a given medication that may be administered at stated intervals if the need for it should arise. The nurse tries to hold off giving the medication, however, for fear the patient might become habituated to it or that he might request it merely because he knows it is available to him. Besides, she may feel that analgesics should be given only after all nursing measures have failed. The patient, aware of the fact that his physician has prescribed a pain-relieving medication for him, and also aware of the fact that he is not receiving it at the designated time, learns to ask for it long before he has any pain. The nurse realizes what he is doing and lets him know, in no uncertain terms, what she thinks of this practice without, however, giving him any kind of assurance that the medication will be forthcoming when the time for it has arrived, or when his pain is such that he really needs the relief-giving drug.

Sometimes, the nurse acts in the opposite manner. The physican may prescribe a pain-relieving medication for a certain patient "in case it is needed," but the busy nurse, trying to keep her patients at a comfort level that will require the minimum amount of work on her part, dispenses it regularly, or even ahead of time, along with the other hundreds of medications she has to distribute at regular intervals. Sometimes, the patient tries to defend himself against this routine and pleads with the nurse to let him have the medicine later when he will really be in need of it. But the nurse does not want to comply, for later on she may be so busy with other matters that she will simply not have time to interrupt what she is doing in order to go through the complicated procedure of unlocking the medicine cabinet, searching for his particular drug, and then charting it in three different places after she has administered it—he will just have to wait until she dispenses the next batch of medications to the entire ward. Upon hearing her explanation, the patient asks that she leave the medicine at his bedside and says that he will either take it when he needs it or he will return it the next day. This request is likely to appear outrageous to the nurse who has been indoctrinated never to leave medications at the patient's bedside, especially medicines that contain narcotics (something that the patient is not supposed to know, of course). Caught on the horns of a dilemma—to take the medicine now when he does not need it, or to not be able to get it later on when he does need it—the patient decides he has no choice but to swallow the pill right then and there.

There is no doubt that the latter kind of incident could be avoided if the nurse did not allow herself to accept such an overwhelming workload that she cannot permit anything to interfere with her desperate attempt to "keep on top of it." The first type of nurse-patient power struggle over pain-relieving drugs can also be prevented if there is reasonably good three-way communication between nurse, patient and physician. It just might be that the patient really does not need the medication as often as the physician has prescribed it, but the physician may not know this. It might also be that the patient asks for an analgesic not because he has pain at the moment, but because he is afraid he will have it unless he keeps himself well medicated. Reassurance by the nurse that medication will be available to him when he needs it may make it possible for him to suffer minor discomfort without adding the burden of a toxic drug to the load already being carried by his severely taxed organism. There are some patients, however, who are so afraid of pain that the fear might be more harmful to them than the effect of the drug itself. Others know from past experience that they have an extremely low tolerance for discomfort and that they are liable to disintegrate emotionally unless they receive early relief from it. Still others have a high tolerance for pain and prefer pain to a state of artificial well-being. And there are those who, as long as they know the reason for their pain, can tolerate it, but who become very anxious if they do not know its cause. Finally, there are patients to whom pain indicates a worsening of their state and who (depending on their relationship to their conditions) may or may not insist that they be kept completely under the influence of drugs.

It should be possible for the nurse to assess a patient's attitude toward pain through observation of his behavior and listening to his comments, and then to proceed accordingly. If the physician permits a certain leeway in the giving of medications, this fact should be utilized in light of the patient's individual needs rather than in light of the nurse's preconceptions about the harmfulness of medications in general or in light of the demands her workload makes on her.

Lack of sleep. Disagreements over sleeping pills frequently proceed along the same lines as those concerning pain-relieving medications. The nurse is often afraid that the patient may become habituated to sedatives and therefore may be reluctant to carry out the physician's p.r.n. orders. Or, in order to get through with her inordinate amount of work, she may try to dispense as many of these drugs as possible within the leeway permitted to her. On the other hand, the patient may have his own ideas about the necessity of sleep and sleep-inducing medications. Thus, a patient for whom sedatives are contraindicated, because he has had an accident to his head or suffers from acute brain damage due to other causes, may nevertheless insist that he be given a sleeping pill. And just because of his brain damage, he may be utterly inaccessible to the explanations offered by the nurse as to why she cannot accede to his request. And so, instead of settling down with the glass of milk and the backrub offered him as a substitute for the pill, he may become increasingly agitated and, in addition, may also prevent his neighbors from getting to sleep. Arguments with such patients are futile, and may only upset them further. If, on the other hand, the nurse asks for a placebo prescription and administers the "medication" with the suggestion that it will make the patient sleep, it will likely do just that.

Fear of dyspnea. Similar power struggles between nurse and patient may center on the matter of mechanical respiratory aids. The patient who has become accustomed to an oscillating bed, a respirator, or to receiving extra oxygen is often reluctant to give up these crutches even though his condition has improved to such an extent that he no longer has any physiological need for them. Frequently, he is anxious and afraid that no one is likely to come to his aid if he should be in trouble, and he wants to insure that his oxygen supply, or whatever he thinks he needs, will not be cut off. An argument based on his improved physiological state misses the point of his concern. Categorically depriving him of his "security blanket" may only upset him to such a degree that he really becomes needful of it. The best way for the nursing staff to proceed is to convey to the patient (not only by words but also by such actions as frequent, unsolicited visits to his room) that he is not abandoned, that they are keeping an eye on him and that, should there be any sign of distress on his part, someone will immediately come to his rescue.

Behavior

In addition to bringing physical factors to the nurse-patient relationship, the patient also brings his behavior. We have referred to the patient's behavior in many contexts throughout this book, particularly in those chapters that deal with the patient's capacity to respond and with his reaction to his condition. Sometimes behavior, instead of being a response to a specific stimulus or situation, is the characteristic manner in which a person deals with most situations he encounters, regardless of whether it is appropriate to the particular situation or not. When we encounter this phenomenon, we are tempted to label the patient according to his predominant pattern of behavior, i.e., we say he is "demanding," "depressed," "suspicious," "hostile," "bizarre," "dependent," and so on.

Habitual behavior. How does the nurse react to behavior that seems to be characteristic for the patient as a person rather than his response to a particular situation? Frequently, she responds to it in one of three ways: in kind; in a manner opposite to that of the patient; or, she may try to withdraw from him altogether. For example, in the case of a patient who is habitually hostile, the nurse may feel her hackles rising every time she meets him and even when she thinks of him in his absence. Or, in trying to protect herself against his perpetual anger, she may find that she is complying with his whims whenever possible, and apologizing profusely when she is not able to comply. On a given day, the patient's hostility may be more than she can bear and as a result, the nurse may find that a headache, a cold or some other physical malaise makes it imperative for her to go off duty at noon.

Some characteristic patient behavior may, in turn, elicit characteristic behaviors from the nurse. For example, the more habitually the patient acts in a dependent manner, the more strongly he is usually urged by the nurse to move toward independence; the more the patients acts in a depressed way, the greater the nurse's efforts to cheer him up; and the more demanding the patient, the more adamant the nurse is likely to be in trying to set limits for him. We are aware of the fact, of course, that the nurse's almost automatic response tends to reinforce the patient's habitual behavior rather than to alter it.

Implications for nursing. What should the nurse do, then? Disregard the patient's behavior altogether or keep herself aloof from it so that she need not react to him in a specific way? No, indeed. Sometimes, the only way one can discover that messages are being conveyed through subtle nuances in the patient's behavior is by noticing one's reactions toward the patient. Thus, the nurse may find herself becoming increasingly irritated toward a patient who cooperates conscientiously with all the rules and regulations of the service and who, if he inadvertently slips up on something, apologizes over and over for his mistake. In itself, i.e., overtly, the patient's behavior should not give rise to irritation. Why, then, does the nurse feel this way? If she takes her own emotional responses seriously, she will be prompted to look more closely at what the patient is doing. She will probably find that her irritation may be in response to a covert message by the patient which asks her to pat him—a 45-year-old man—on the head for having been "a good boy"; or it may be in response to a concealed message of "I am a good soldier" mockery.

Knowing what it is about the patient's behavior that irritates her may give her some idea about his motivation. It does not necessarily imply that she should share her ideas and feelings on this matter with the patient, however. Whether she does this would depend, first of all, upon the patient's readiness to hear what she might have to say. It would also depend on the nurse's ability to convey her feelings to the patient more as a request for his validation of what she thinks he is trying to communicate to her than as an expression of her emotions. Thus, she might ask him, "Are you trying to let me know that you deserve praise for sticking exactly to the rules?" or "Are you, perhaps, trying to make fun of all the rules and regulations the staff here is imposing upon you?" Whether to approach the patient about her feelings toward him would depend, finally, upon the nurse's ability to cope with his probable response, for no one cares to have his habitual behaviors scrutinized and almost everyone will, at least in the beginning, defend them angrily. Yet, many people *are* willing to look at their behavior and to reevaluate it when necessary if, at the same time, they are sustained by the sincere concern of the person who challenges it.

If the nurse finds it impossible to confront the patient with his covert message, maybe because she feels that she does not possess enough skill or that she has not yet established a sufficiently stable relationship with him, she should suggest that someone who is less irritated by his behavior than she is, take care of him.

In any case, however, it should be possible for the nurse to become aware that she is responding automatically to patients' habitual behaviors and that she stop doing this. Again, this is easier said than done, for many nurses are convinced that patients should not act the way they do but rather the way nurses think they ought to act. The reason for this, of course, is that nurses are often insufficiently aware of their own value systems (*see* Chapter 1). Here, it suffices to say, that, as the nurse becomes more aware of her own value system, she will become increasingly more tolerant of patients' habitual behaviors and will also find it increasingly easier to sense the messages they are trying to convey.

Habitual behaviors, though not often useful in actual situations, do perform certain functions for the patient. They may represent an effort to cope with his condition or an attempt to negotiate a certain phase in it. This is frequently the case with an excessively demanding or dependent patient who is trying to conceal from himself and others that he is afraid of his condition, or that it has overwhelmed him and he is unable to cope with it. If the nurse can pick up the messages which are contained in the patient's behavior, she will find a way of helping the patient with the actual problem rather than having to fight the behavior itself.

Behavior as a personality trait. Sometimes the patient's habitual behavior indicates a personality trait which he had long before he was ill and will probably still exhibit long after he has become well. Besides being to some extent inherited, any personality trait a patient may have has also served the function of helping the patient (or his personality) to survive in very difficult situations when he was young. Later, after his life situation changed, this trait may have served as a barrier rather than as an aid to his subsequent adaptations. But this is really his problem, and except perhaps in the clinical area of psychiatry, is not usually the problem for which he has been placed under the nurse's care. It may help both the nurse and the patient, therefore, if the nurse can take his personality trait, (i.e., his habitual behavior) for granted in the same way she would take his physical traits for granted. In this way, she will be able to protect a patient who is, say, lacking in flexibility, from excessive environmental stresses just as she would protect a patient who lacks skin pigment from excessive exposure to the sun. She will structure such a patient's day to the best of her ability and will inform him of his routine beforehand. If unforeseen changes in routines must occur, she will inform him of these changes and give him an opportunity to ventilate his annoyance.

Similarly, instead of pushing a very dependent patient toward independence, the nurse may suggest to him that someone will be available to look after him until he can again take care of himself. Or, if the patient is likely to become hostile when he is frightened, she can keep his hostility to a minimum if instead of reprimanding him for his attitude, she subtly allays his fears by letting him ask questions or by offering some explanatory statements of her own.

How well the nurse will be able to accept the patient's habitual behavior and to structure his environment around it, will depend upon her understanding of the purposes that a particular personality trait serves, in general, and for a given patient. In other words it will help her to understand that behavior, as well as illness, usually follows certain natural laws. It, too, has an etiology and is brought into being by a sequence of predisposing and precipitating factors. The sequence of predisposing factors is sometimes called the *generic* cause of the behavior, and that of the precipitating ones is called the *dynamic* cause. The nurse will do well to build an arsenal of knowledge around the generic and precipitating factors of those habitual behaviors which she is most likely to encounter.

Resentment. This type of behavior is often seen in long-term patients. What are some of the predisposing factors that might lead a person to become resentful? Usually, there has been an early home situation in which the person was exposed to behavior by others that made him very angry, but he was not allowed to express his anger for fear of punishment or loss of love. As a result, he never learned to express anger openly, but would respond to anyone who provoked it with a smoldering, lingering, half-suppressed antagonism.

A person who has a tendency toward resentment is likely to respond this way whenever he has real or imagined reason to be afraid of authority figures or of losing the love of someone on whom he is, in some way, dependent. The hospital setting that puts the patient in a particularly dependent situation will naturally accentuate this tendency. Not only is he almost completely stripped of his autonomy and must submit to doctor's orders and ward regulations, but he is also much aware of how dependent he is upon the staff, particularly if he is immobilized in some way. Even when he is annoyed by something that occurs, he does not dare express his annoyance openly. And so, instead of dissipating itself through expression, his annoyance lingers on, in spite of his efforts to hide it. Often, the effect of this on the staff is that they withdraw, at least partially, from the patient, or unconsciously try to rub the patient the wrong way, perhaps so that the flame of anger can burst out into the open.

If the nurse is aware of the probable generic and dynamic etiology of the patient's behavior and the sequential steps that have probably led up to it, there is a possibility that she can help the patient overcome his tendency toward resentment. Naturally, she cannot aim to change the patient's past. This, and his resulting tendencies to behave in a certain way, have become part and parcel of his personality. She can, however, help him adjust to his current situation. Knowing—or at least having a good hunch—that the patient has a fear of authority figures and also fears of loss of love, should he show anger, the nurse, for one, can act as permissibly toward him as is feasible. She can go out of her way to accept his gestures of resentment as an expression of actual anger, and indicate to him through her words and her actual non-punitive behavior that she understands why someone in his position might be angry. In addition, she can demonstrate to him by repeated examples, that even though he is angry, she will not neglect his care; that, in fact, his nursing care is quite independent of his being friendly or unfriendly toward his nurse. It is likely that before long he will learn to express his anger more openly. At first, he may well over-correct his tendency to suppress his anger and, consequently, will express it more forcefully than would someone who is used to telling others when he is annoyed. If the nurse can take this as a stage in the patient's learning and refrain from retaliating in kind, reprimanding the patient or otherwise showing her disapproval, he may soon learn to find a way to express his anger by communicating what he has to say without offending his listeners. It is important, of course, that the other members of the nursing staff be informed of the patient's problem area and that they, too, be helped to deal with it judiciously, for if he is punished along the way, he will merely be confirmed in his position and will retreat again into his fortress of resentment—perhaps forever.

Naturally, it is not always possible for the nurse to make use of her knowledge to her own best advantage and that of her patient. Frequently the patient's behavior, his symptom, his appearance, or his value system—in light of his age or his cultural background—may be such that the nurse reacts to it almost instinctively and hence finds it impossible to disengage herself from the situation enough to let her knowledge come into play. If, however, she is fortunate enough to have access to a resource person who, while accepting the nurse's emotional reaction, can at the same time remind her of what she knows apart from the way she feels, the nurse will usually be able to move out of the impasse.

Let us hope that before long every nurse practicing in a clinical area will have access to someone to whom she may turn for help; someone to whom she will feel free to reveal her difficulties and who will not violate her confidence; someone who can help her to solve each particular situation so that she will learn from it, not only for the situation at hand but also for future, similar occasions; someone who, in other words, can contribute to the nurse's continued professional growth.

Suggested Readings

American Academy of Pediatrics. *Care of Children in Hospitals.* Chicago, Ill.: American Academy of Pediatrics, 1960.

American Nurses' Association. *Code of Ethics.* New York: American Nurses' Association, 1950, revised 1960.

Ayllon, Teodoro, and Michael, Jack. "The Psychiatric Nurse as a Behavioral Engineer," *Jour. of Exp. Anal. Behavior 2* (Oct., 1959), pp. 323-334.

Blake, Florence. *The Child, His Parents and the Nurse.* Philadelphia: J. B. Lippincott Co., 1954.

Blake, Florence. *Open Heart Surgery in Children.* Washington, D. C.: Department of Health, Education and Welfare, 1964.

Blumberg, Jeanne E., and Drummond, Eleanor E. *Nursing Care of the Long-Term Patient.* New York: Springer Publishing Co., 1963.

Cattell, Raymond, and Scheier, I. H. *Meaning and Measurement of Neuroticism and Anxiety.* New York: Ronald Press, 1961.

Erickson, Florence. "The Nurse in Modern Pediatrics," *International Journal of Nursing Studies 2* (1965), pp. 139-144.

Feifel, Herman (ed.). *The Meaning of Death.* New York: McGraw-Hill Book Co., 1959.

Friedenberg, Edgar. *Coming of Age in America.* New York: Random House, 1965.

Hammar, S. L., and Eddy, J. K. *Nursing Care of the Adolescent.* New York: Springer Publishing Co., 1966.

Hollingshead, August B., and Redlich, Frederick. *Social Class and Mental Illness.* New York: John Wiley & Sons, 1958.

Langner, Thomas S., and Michael, Stanley T. *Life Stress and Mental Health, II.* Glencoe, Ill.: The Free Press, 1963.

Lazarus, Richard S. *Psychological Stress and the Coping Process.* New York: McGraw-Hill Book Co., 1966.

Lewin, Kurt. *Resolving Social Conflicts.* New York: Harper and Bros., 1948.

Maier, Henry W. *Three Theories of Child Development.* New York: Harper and Row, 1965.

Marlow, Dorothy R. *Textbook of Pediatric Nursing* (2nd ed.). Philadelphia: W. B. Saunders Co., 1965.

Opler, Marvin K. *Culture and Social Psychiatry.* New York: Atherton Press, 1967.

Plank, Emma. *Working With Children in Hospitals.* Cleveland, Ohio: Western Reserve University Press, 1962.

Shore, Milton F. (ed.). *Red is the Color of Hurting.* Washington, D. C.: National Clearing House for Mental Health Information, 1967.

Skipper, James K., and Leonard, Robert C. *Social Interaction and Patient Care.* Philadelphia: J. B. Lippincott Co., 1965.

Srole, Leo *et al. Mental Health in the Metropolis.* McGraw-Hill Book Co., 1962.

Ujhely, Gertrud B. "The Aged Problem Patient in the General Hospital" and "On the Ability to Be of Help." Unpublished papers.

Vernon, David *et al. The Psychological Responses of Children to Hospitalization and Illness.* Springfield, Ill.: Charles C Thomas, 1965.

Wu, Ruth. "Explaining Treatments to Young Children," *American Journal of Nursing* 65 (July, 1965), pp. 71-73.

Index

E

F

J

K

L

M

N

O

P

S

T

U